I0082460

Neurohacking
For
Online Learning

Study and Life Habits Optimized for Your
Personal Mind-Body Energy State

Robert Keith Wallace, PhD, Carol Paredes, MS

© Copyright 2023 by Robert Keith Wallace and Carol Paredes
Printed in the United States of America
No part of this publication may be reproduced, stored in a retrieval system, or transmitted in any form or by any means, electronic, mechanical, photocopying, recording, or otherwise, without prior written permission of the publisher.

Transcendental Meditation®, TM®, Maharishi®, Maharishi International University®, MIU®, and Maharishi AyurVeda® are protected trademarks and are used in the US under license or with permission.

The advice and information in this book relates to health care and should be used to supplement rather than to replace the advice of your doctor or trained health professional. If you have any serious, acute, or chronic health concerns, please consult a trained health professional who can fully assess your needs and address them effectively.

The publisher and authors disclaim liability for any medical outcomes as a result of applying any of the methods discussed in this book.

ISBN 978-1-7357401-7-1

Library of Congress Control Number 2023912606

DharmaPublications.com

Dharma Publications, Fairfield, IA

To Our Very Dear Children and Grandchildren

OTHER BOOKS BY

Robert Keith Wallace

16 Biohack for Longevity
Shortcuts to a Healthier, Happier, Longer Life
Robert Keith Wallace, PhD, Ted Wallace, MS, Samantha Wallace

Living in Balance with Maharishi AyurVeda
Practical Therapies for Consciousness-Based Health
Robert Keith Wallace, PhD, Karin Pirc, MD, Julia Clarke, MS

Self Empower
Using Self Coaching, Neuroadaptability, and Ayurveda
Robert Keith Wallace, PhD, Samantha Wallace,
Ted Wallace, MS

Trouble in Paradise
How to Deal with People Who Push Your Buttons
Using Total Brain Coaching
Robert Keith Wallace, PhD, Samantha Wallace,
Ted Wallace, MS

The Coherence Code
How to Maximize Your Performance and Success in Business
For Individuals, Teams, and Organizations
Robert Keith Wallace, PhD, Ted Wallace, MS,
Samantha Wallace

Total Brain Coaching
A Holistic System of Effective Habit Change
For the Individual, Team, and Organization
Ted Wallace, MS, Robert Keith Wallace, PhD,
Samantha Wallace

The Rest and Repair Diet
Heal Your Gut, Improve Your Physical and Mental Health,
and Lose Weight
Robert Keith Wallace, PhD, Samantha Wallace,
Andrew Stenberg, MA, Jim Davis, DO, and Alexis Farley

Gut Crisis
How Diet, Probiotics, and Friendly Bacteria
Help You Lose Weight and Heal Your Body and Mind
Robert Keith Wallace, PhD, Samantha Wallace

Dharma Parenting
Understand Your Child's Brilliant Brain
for Greater Happiness, Health, Success, and Fulfillment
Robert Keith Wallace, PhD, Frederick Travis, PhD

Quantum Golf
The Path to Golf Mastery
REVISED Second Edition
Kjell Enhager, Robert Keith Wallace, PhD, Samantha Wallace

An Introduction to Transcendental Meditation
Improve Your Brain Functioning, Create Ideal Health,
and Gain Enlightenment Naturally, Easily, Effortlessly
Robert Keith Wallace, PhD, Lincoln Akin Norton

Transcendental Meditation
A Scientist's Journey to Happiness, Health, and Peace
Robert Keith Wallace, PhD

The Neurophysiology of Enlightenment
How the Transcendental Meditation and TM-Sidhi Program
Transform the Functioning of the Human Body
Robert Keith Wallace, PhD

Maharishi Ayurveda and Vedic Technology
Creating Ideal Health for the Individual and World
Robert Keith Wallace, PhD

The Coherence Effect
Tapping into the Laws of Nature that Govern Health,
Happiness, and Higher Brain Functioning
Robert Keith Wallace, PhD, Jay B. Marcus,
Christopher S. Clark, MD

CONTENTS

CHAPTER 1

UNLEASHING THE MIND'S POTENTIAL

Welcome to neurohacking—a journey through the enigmatic landscape of the mind that promises to unlock the true potential of the human brain.

What lies beneath the intriguing term neurohacking? Traditional hacking usually involves the manipulation of a computer's software. Neurohacking involves the ability to shape the brain's software and hardware.

Consider the fact that each experience we undergo has the power to rewire the brain. Every encounter, every sensation, shapes the delicate architecture of our brains. This constant change is akin to the brushstrokes of an artist, as our experiences paint an ever-changing portrait on our innermost world. What if we could harness this power and rewire our neural pathways to direct the course of our own evolution? This is the essence of neurohacking—a practice that merges the realms of science and personal transformation.

Let's first consider the practice of meditation. We will talk specifically about Transcendental Meditation (TM), since that has been Keith's focus of research for over fifty years. When you practice TM you are doing an ancient form of neurohacking that rewires your brain and improves many aspects of your life. These include both your mental and physical health, as well as creativity and your ability to learn. These findings have been documented by numerous scientific studies.

Online Learning

What else can you do to improve your ability to learn? Online courses can be daunting. You are asked to comprehend and retain knowledge while engaged in the demands of everyday life. You may have a job or a family to take care of—all while you are absorbing new concepts and skills. We will examine a number of neurohacks that can help you manage the challenges of online learning. Remember that these neurohacks will only be useful to you if you are able to do them regularly and turn them into habits.

There is a distinction between neurohacks and habits. Neurohacks are attempts or experiments to improve the functioning of your brain through some modern or ancient practice such as meditation.

Habits are routines stored in your brain as ingrained neural circuits. Take, for instance, the process of learning to ride a bicycle. Initially this new skill demands focused attention and the activity of many parts of the brain that have to be highly coordinated. Gradually the process evolves into an almost instinctive activity requiring minimal conscious thought and brain activity. Habits conserve energy. When we practice TM, for example, regularly twice a day over an extended period, transcending naturally becomes a habit. We don't have to expend any energy thinking about doing it. Through sustained repetition, a neuro-hack gradually evolves into a habit.

Think of learning a new habit as creating a new pathway in your brain, a pathway over which information can travel easily with minimum effort. Some habits are good for our lives while others such as smoking, excess drinking, and drug use can have a negative impact. The easiest way to eliminate a bad habit is to create a new habit. The creation of a new habit is like construct-ing a fresh neural highway, paving the way for ever more refined transformation.

Habits shape the network of our mind. Through repetition and practice, the physical neural pathways used in a habit so-lidify, enabling us to navigate life's obstacles with effortless pre-cision. The brain has a remarkable form of adaptability called neuroplasticity. With every new experience there is a dance of involved neurons and all their delicate parts as they rewire themselves in response to the changes in our inner and outer environment, shaping our thoughts, emotions, and actions. The brain is especially dynamic when we are young and learning new skills and knowledge but this dance of the neurons continues even as we get older. We are all capable of changing ourselves from within, changing the physical network of our billions of neurons. The possibilities are limitless.

The Structure of Habits

One of the classic books on habits is *The Power of Habit* by Charles Duhigg. He explains why habits exist and how they can be modified. He uses stories from all areas of life, ranging from the board rooms of Procter and Gamble, to the sidelines of the NFL, to the front lines of the civil rights movement. At its core, *The Power of Habit*, gives us a clear understanding of the basic components of habits. Understanding these elements and how to make best use of them will enable us to adopt healthy habits more easily, whether they be exercising regularly, drinking enough water, or doing our homework on time.

The graphic below displays the basic parts of the habit loop.

Golden rule of habit change:
"Keep the Cue and Reward, replace the Routine."

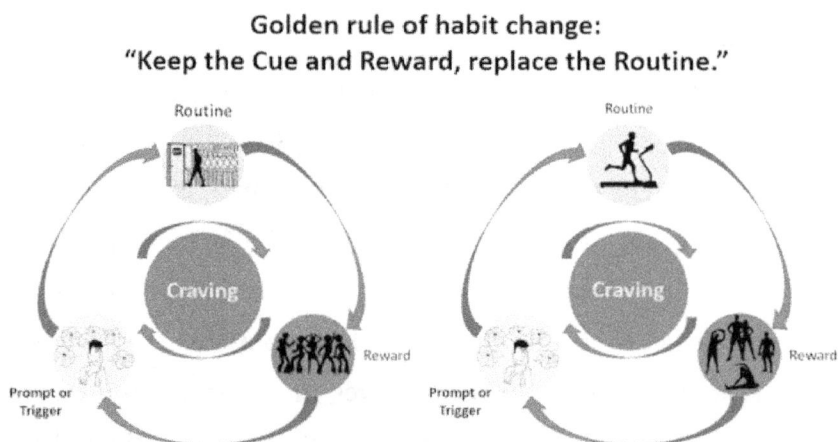

Most of us have some sort of craving. The craving might be very subtle. You might not even notice it, but it's usually activated by a prompt or a trigger of some kind. Once this trigger occurs, it causes you to follow a routine. If you get a reward for that activity, it is reinforced and you keep on repeating it over and over again.

An example of this might relate to your studies. You are about to put your attention on studying, but as you pass the kitchen you feel a desire to eat something. This anticipation of a pleasant reward from eating causes you to put off your attempt to start your homework.

How do you change such a process? Duhigg suggests that you don't try to change the trigger or reward. Instead change the routine. One way to do this might be to start chewing a piece of gum (if you like gum) instead of eating. The act of putting something in your mouth and having it full of flavor satisfies that desire. Now you can go and finish your homework. By changing your stimulus-response routine, you also created a new reward—the sense of accomplishment in finishing your paper and being able to modify your behavior. You can go one step further and find new prompts or triggers that will help you remember to start your homework. Now you are learning the mechanics of how to create a new habit.

Study Habits

When it comes to doing your homework, one powerful habit is to establish a specific time or day dedicated to your finishing your assignments. Life can be hectic for all of us, and without a designated schedule, important tasks like homework can easily slip away. We know that homework isn't always the most enjoyable activity, and many students are often tempted to procrastinate until the last moment. By designating a particular day like

"Homework Monday," and safeguarding it for your academic endeavors throughout your educational journey, you create a weekly routine structure that ensures consistent progress. To assist with time management, you can set reminders on your phone to alert you when it's time to study or engage in your learning routine. For example, if you find it most effective to study at 7 p.m. every night, setting a reminder will help you prioritize your learning goals and stay on track.

Learning in the company of others can also be a valuable approach. Joining study groups or finding a study buddy provides an opportunity for collaborative learning and mutual support. Having someone to discuss concepts with and help clarify doubts can enhance your understanding and retention of the material. Additionally, seeking guidance from a mentor or teaching assistant can provide valuable insights and expertise. Remember, never hesitate to ask questions. No question is ever foolish, and seeking clarity is a crucial part of the learning journey.

Embrace the mindset that you are a "good learner" . Don't shy away from seeking the knowledge you need. Sometimes, understanding certain concepts or information may be challenging, and it's essential to recognize that it's not your fault if you are confused. The delivery method of information plays a significant role in comprehension. If you find yourself struggling to grasp a concept, don't hesitate to express your confusion. Raise your hand and say, "I don't get it." This shift in perspective allows you to share the responsibility of acquiring new knowledge with the instructor, rather than putting the blame solely on yourself. Remember, learning is a partnership between the teacher and the student, and it's crucial to advocate for your understanding. If needed, seek assistance from a life coach or mentor who can provide guidance and support.

Turning the Page

In moments of frustration or mental fatigue, there is a powerful technique I (Carol) call "Turning the Page." Here is a personal anecdote from my own experience. As a child, I had a set of encyclopedias—a treasure trove of knowledge spanning from A to Z. One day, I observed my father reading them from cover to cover. Intrigued, I asked him, "Isn't that boring?" With a twinkle in his eye, he replied, "You just turn the page. They're not all boring." Little did I know that this seemingly simple advice would become a profound lesson in my journey of learning.

Years later, while studying programming, I encountered moments of disinterest, confusion, and fatigue. On one occasion, during a flight, I found myself reading the same paragraph repeatedly, struggling to grasp the concepts. Exhausted, I was ready to give up. Then, a whisper echoed in my mind—my father's voice urging me to "just turn the page." And so, I did. I released the anxiety and frustration associated with that page, and continued reading. As I progressed, around page 150, a remarkable shift occurred. The pieces began to align, and clarity washed over me. By letting go and persevering, I overcame my mental block and continued to absorb knowledge with renewed vigor.

"Turning the Page" serves as a powerful approach to manage anxiety and maintain progress in the face of challenge. When a task or concept overwhelms you, take a step back, breathe deeply, and shift your focus. Remind yourself that it's just one page, one step. Keep moving forward. Taking breaks, going for a walk, or engaging in relaxing activities can also alleviate stress and reinvigorate your mind. By adopting this mindset, you can conquer obstacles and embrace the learning process with resilience and determination.

Another effective strategy in forming new habits is breaking them down into simple steps. This approach proved invaluable during my programming studies. When faced with the daunting task of mastering an entire textbook before an exam, I divided it into manageable sections. Each week, I focused on a specific portion, further dividing it into daily study goals. By breaking the material into bite-sized pieces, the overwhelming book transformed into a series of small, achievable targets. To reinforce the habit, I established triggers, such as studying every morning at 7 a.m., aligning the task with my natural inclination as a morning person. I also introduced rewards to celebrate my progress, including visually tracking my advancement through the book with a colorful, fun bookmark. This combination of breaking tasks down and establishing a routine with triggers and rewards propelled me toward my learning goals.

In summary, the lessons of "Turning the Page" and breaking habits into simple components hold immense value in our pursuit of knowledge. By applying these techniques, we can navigate the challenges of learning, manage our anxiety, and cultivate habits that lead to meaningful progress. Remember, the journey of learning is a transformative experience, and with the right insights and tools, you possess the means to unlock your full potential.

Four Components

Let's explore the four components involved in neurohacking your learning cycle, which are:

1. Motivate

2. Personalize

3. Experiment

4. Be Real

We can use the example of reading a textbook and identify each of these components. The first is Motivate, which came through my father's encouragement of "Turning the Page". We will delve into the basis of motivation in greater detail in future lessons. The second component, Personalize, was illustrated in my preference for numbers and analytical tools to track my progress. This approach certainly won't hold the same attraction for everyone. Understanding how to personalize your learning methods can greatly benefit you and equip you with powerful tools. The third component, Experiment, came when I applied my father's wisdom in my own work. I had an open mind and tried what my father told me. If something doesn't work initially, that's okay. Experiment again and find approaches that work for you. In my case, I found that "Turning the Page" worked. The fourth component, Be Real, was validated by how it helped me get through my work and that in itself was a reward. We will thoroughly explore each of these four components because a deeper understanding of how to neurohack the learning cycle helps you to more easily adopt new healthy learning habits.

You may encounter many challenges in your learning journey. It's important to recognize that pursuing a degree takes time, ranging from two to several years. Whether you engage in online or classroom learning, there will always be challenges. In a traditional classroom, you have dedicated learning time and minimal distractions. However, with online learning, you must navigate many video and live lectures and find suitable time slots to watch them. They may not fit neatly into your current routine.

To overcome these obstacles, it is crucial to create an environment that is conducive to learning. Designate a specific study space in your home where you can focus and minimize interruptions. Turn off devices, such as your phone, and prioritize uninterrupted study time. Even dedicating 30 or 40 minutes to focused study can yield substantial knowledge and enhance your sense of accomplishment. Additionally, you should anticipate other potential hurdles that life may present. Planning and being prepared to adapt are keys to overcoming difficult situations. Successful individuals view challenges as opportunities for growth and problem-solving.

To help you develop new habits, we will provide you with a toolkit. By identifying your current personal habits and understanding the challenges specific to online learning, you can make adjustments to both your internal and external environments. We will explore various techniques for enhancing both learning and overall well-being. For example, when you learn Transcendental Meditation, you are learning to regulate your nervous system and positively rewire your brain.

Stress and Learning

Take a few moments and reflect on your current obstacles to learning and studying. Consider various factors such as your environment, sleep patterns, or work commitments. Additionally, write down any experiences where emotions or stress have impacted your ability to learn effectively. Our task will be to help you to find practical ways to resolve these situations, to create greater internal stability and happiness, and to provide specific guidance for your online learning experience.

Dr. Andrew Huberman, an associate professor of neurobiology at Stanford, has some very interesting observations about learning. He's an expert in various behavioral areas, such as fear and courage and is a popular neuroscientist who believes that his spreading of knowledge on Instagram is equally as important as his publishing articles in prestigious journals like *Nature* and

Scientific American. He's passionate about making neuroscience accessible to the world.

Dr. Huberman explains three key factors that enhance our understanding and learning. First, he emphasizes the importance of lowering our internal sense of urgency and remaining calm. This helps us to absorb information effectively. Currently, with everyone caught up in a frenzy, our collective consciousness seems to be losing focus. Dr. Huberman suggests finding ways to deactivate the amygdala circuits that are responsible for our fight-or-flight response. He believes it's crucial to teach future generations how to regulate their nervous systems. By recognizing a surge of adrenaline as a compromised state, we can prioritize calmness as a prerequisite for listening and learning. Dr. Huberman argues that we should begin by learning physiological self-regulation. Although he doesn't have a definitive plan for achieving this, his dedication to teaching neuroscience on Instagram reflects his belief that our individual ability to regulate ourselves is fundamental to our cultural advancement.

Dr. Huberman's insights on self-regulation align with the techniques we will be teaching you. Simple practices like "Turning the Page" and breaking assignments into manageable chunks help to alleviate anxiety and enhance focus. Transcendental Meditation is another powerful tool to improve self-regulation. This practice can be done individually or in a group, and it effectively regulates the physiology, calms our inner state, and improves learning abilities. Dr. Huberman also discusses other fascinating approaches, such as the benefits of sunlight, which we'll explore in a future lesson. By learning new techniques for both learning and life, you can lower your stress level, increase your energy, enhance your focus, and unfold the full potential of your brain and consciousness.

CHAPTER 2

UNDERSTANDING MOTIVATION

What drives your desire to learn? Is it fear? Is it inspiration? Fear is generally unpleasant, but for some people fear of failure can be a powerful motivator. On the other hand, most of us thrive on inspiration, enjoying mental stimulation and the opportunity to engage in creative endeavors. Motivation is essential because it is closely tied to our deep-rooted beliefs and identity. What does it means to motivate yourself?

There are many underlying factors, some internal and some external, which cause us to move forward toward our goals. We all have basic needs and desires such as for food, shelter, and safety. We also have higher goals for love, belongingness, and becoming the best version of ourselves.

Setting Goals

Setting a goal is often a fundamental tool in motivating yourself. In his book *Atomic Habits*, James Clear provides an example from *Alice in Wonderland*. When Alice asks the Cheshire Cat which way to go, the cat responds, "That depends a good deal on where you want to get to." This seemingly simple interaction holds significant meaning. It helps if you have a clear intention and know where you want to go and what you want to accomplish. The clearer your intention, the easier it becomes to prioritize your desires and allocate your energy most effectively. Once you establish a goal, such as aiming for an A in a particular class, it can be a powerful driving force that propels you toward success.

Motivation can be driven by rewards. There are internal rewards such as the joy, satisfaction, and the sense of accomplishment we experience from engaging in a particular activity. There are also external rewards, such as recognition, praise, money, or other benefits that fuel us to do more. If we look deeper inside ourselves, we will find that we are ultimately motivated by our beliefs and values, which give us a sense of purpose in life. Motivation can give us a feeling of self-empowerment, a feeling that we can make a difference. This is reinforced when we have encouragement from our friends, family, and community. Finally, motivation is influenced by our past successes. If we have had wins, even small wins, this can give us the confidence to move forward.

When I (Carol) first entered the technology field many years ago, I had a strong desire to go beyond being a systems engineer. I wanted to become the engineer who could teach and inspire other engineers. This goal filled me with motivation and enthusiasm. I wanted to make a significant impact and overcome the challenges of being a woman in a predominantly male industry. Building leadership and integrity was also important to me.

I have previously mentioned two goals that I had in my own life. One was breaking down a book and committing to reading a specific number of pages each day. Although it was a small goal, it ultimately contributed to the larger goal of completing the book on time, which then led to the accomplishment of an even larger goal of preparing for an exam that was weeks away. These tangible goals gave me direction and purpose.

What I didn't mention earlier was that I gave myself a five-year timeframe to achieve my ultimate goal (be an engineer who teaches other engineers). I cut that larger goal into smaller actionable steps: determining what subjects to study, identifying which tests to pass, and so on. By keeping this larger goal on the horizon, I remained focused and energized.

It's important to note that even when circumstances caused me to adjust my timeline, such as the passing of my dear father, I still kept my goal in sight. I may have needed to adapt and extend the timeline slightly, but the important element was having a defined goal to work toward. Setting goals, both short-term and long-term, plays a vital role in maintaining motivation and propelling us forward.

It's interesting to note that goals can vary in their nature. On the one hand, you can have simple and concrete goals, such as allocating 15 minutes each day at 8 a.m. to complete your homework. Such a goal is specific and easily measurable. On the other hand, you may have more abstract goals, like improving your learning ability or experiencing higher states of consciousness.

When I (Keith) first started practicing meditation, my goal

was to establish a habit of meditating twice a day, so I could gain the maximum benefits without needing to consciously think about it. During this time, I was fortunate enough to have an opportunity to be with Maharishi Mahesh Yogi, the founder of the Transcendental Meditation Technique. His words and teachings were incredibly inspiring and powerful, leading me to adopt the abstract, but nevertheless deep, goal of pursuing enlightenment. It is important to have both abstract and concrete goals. Abstract goals serve to elevate and inspire us, taking us to higher levels of motivation, while concrete goals provide clear and tangible targets for our action.

Think about your motivations. What goal do you have in mind? Why did you choose this goal? What keeps you excited and drives you? Once you have identified some of your goals, it becomes essential to prioritize them. In the chart on the next page you can observe a person stating multiple aspirations in the left column: being a straight-A student, maintaining a healthy diet, prioritizing family, and playing well in a volleyball league.

While all of these goals are commendable, it is crucial to determine which goals hold greater priority for the individual to apply their energy effectively. In the right column, the individual has placed her family as her top priority, followed by studying. A university student might prioritize being a straight-A student first and then their family. It depends on each person's values and circumstances.

NEED TO PRIORITIZE GOALS

Goals	Prioritize
I want to be a straight A student.	1. I want to take care of my family first.
I want to eat well and avoid junk foods.	2. I want to be a straight A student.
I want to take care of my family first.	3. I want to exercise everyday and be a star in my volleyball league.
I want to exercise everyday and be a star in my volleyball league.	4. I want to eat well and avoid junk foods.

Consider another example. Suppose your goals are to exercise daily, become a star in your volleyball league, eat well, and avoid junk food. If these were my priorities, I (Carol) would prioritize eating well and avoiding junk food as the first step. This is because maintaining a healthy diet is vital for giving me the energy to play volleyball. I would focus on exercising every day to enhance my performance and achieve my goal of becoming a star player.

The next key is to personalize your goals. See if they align with your deeper values in life. In a later chapter we will go through this process in detail. It is important to remember that we need to start with small doable steps. James Clear introduces the concept of atomic habits, referring to small and simple actions. He emphasizes the importance of solving life's challenges with minimal energy and effort. As he says,

> The ultimate purpose of habits is to solve the problems of life with as little energy and effort as possible.

He presents four ideas to cultivate effective habits. Make them:

- obvious
- attractive
- easy
- satisfying

Identity-Based Habits

One of the central ideas in his book is identity-based habits. A student might hold onto beliefs like, "I'm not good at studying," or, "I've never been successful in this area." These are assumed identities that may not even be true. Clear recommends consciously creating an identity for yourself that is positive and comprehensive. Try letting go of any old limiting identities and instead affirm a positive identity. For instance, you can say to yourself, "I am a very intelligent person," or "I am a great student," or "I love to study." By assuming these identities, you will notice a shift in your thinking, as well as your approach to studying, and to your overall life. Consider writing down your chosen identity on a piece of paper and placing it somewhere visible in your room. Start embodying that identity and observe the changes it brings to your mindset, study habits, and every aspect of your life.

There are three layers to any behavior change, according to Clear. The first is the outcome. For example, your outcome might be to finish your homework on time. The second layer is the process. This involves the way in which you achieve your desired outcome. Are you dedicating study time each week and protecting that time as an important part of your life? A process often involves creating a specific routine. To achieve your desired outcome more efficiently, sometimes you must change old habits and adopt new ones.

Many people, for example, have a habit of immediately checking their emails or engaging with social media when they turn on their computers or phones. This is understandable because their device offers a form of social interaction and communication. However, if you want to prioritize your own tasks, such as completing homework, it's important to set aside a specific time period for it and make it a sacred commitment. By establishing a dedicated and scheduled time for your homework, you can develop a habit where it becomes the first thing you do. Initially, it may take some time to adjust, but with persistence, you can make prioritizing homework a natural routine. Consider finishing the task as a reward to yourself—by completing your homework first, you can then indulge in checking emails or social media later.

In this way, you ensure that your own tasks and goals receive the full attention they deserve before you attend to either social media or external obligations. While studying may not be inherently enjoyable for everyone, treating it as a priority and creating a pleasant study environment can make it a lot more manageable, less stressful, and more rewarding. By dedicating time and establishing a process, you can effectively change your habits to achieve your desired outcome.

The third layer of behavior change is identity. This layer

involves transforming your beliefs and self-image. By consciously adopting the mindset of being a top student and embracing this new worldview, you can experience remarkable transformation. Your thoughts and beliefs have a powerful influence on your actions and behaviors.

When you internalize the identity of being a top student and genuinely believe in it, you'll begin to notice a significant difference. Your mind and body work in harmony, and you'll begin to align your actions with that identity. It's astonishing how your mere choice to assume this identity can shape your behavior and propel you toward becoming the student you aspire to be.

Simon Sinek, a renowned business consultant, introduced a similar idea called The Golden Circle. At the outer edge of the circle is the "what, " which in the case of a company, is the products they produce. The next layer is labeled "how." Every company knows their goods or services, while some also know "how" they are different from other companies. Finally, at the inner core of the circle lies the identity or the "why" behind the company's actions. Sinek feels that very few companies are aware of why they do what they do. He says the why is not about profit or the exit strategy. It has to do with purpose or belief. He explains that all the inspired leaders think from the inside out. They all start with why. For instance, Apple computer has the slogan "Think Different." The way Apple challenges the current level of thinking is by designing beautiful products, making them simple and user friendly. They have a clear identity, a clear purpose upon which all other actions are based.

Who do you want to be? Craft your identity based on your deepest desires. Reinforce this identity by attaining small wins. Experiment with micro neurohacks. If they work, then solidify them as regular habits. Once you experience one accomplishment, it becomes easier to achieve further success.

When I (Carol) was studying to become a software engineer, I set a goal for myself: passing the 12 required exams to become a Microsoft Certified System Engineer (MCSE) on two different operating platforms. Each exam became a small win on my path to achieving my main goal. My confidence grew with each exam I passed, and I felt a sense of accomplishment. It was this series of small wins that propelled me toward my ultimate goal of becoming an engineer and teaching others in the field.

Not everyone will receive an "A" grade on every assignment. The purpose of education is not solely to achieve top grades but mainly to learn and gain knowledge. Strive to be the best student you can be and embrace the learning process. Receiving a lower grade like a "B" or a "C" indicates that there are areas where you can further improve your understanding or expression. Making mistakes is natural and part of the learning journey.

When I first owned a computer, I accidentally erased everything on it, including the operating system. Despite the initial setback, I quickly learned how to reinstall everything and even became proficient enough to assist others with their computer issues. I share this anecdote to emphasize the value of mistakes and the learning opportunities they offer.

Make a conscious decision to be the best student you can be.

Remember, perfection is not the goal, rather focus on continuous improvement. Keep track of your small wins along the way. You may choose to record them somewhere, such as collecting gold stars on a bulletin board. These small wins accumulate and contribute to your overall progress. By assuming the identity of someone who strives for excellence, you can embrace your mistakes as valuable learning experiences; they provide insights that contribute to your growth. Remember, some of the strategies that work for me today stem from mistakes I made in the past.

Consider the various factors that drive your motivation, such as obtaining a new skill or being the first in your family to earn a college degree. Reflect on your goals, whether it's submitting all assignments on time or protecting your dedicated study time. Your formula for success consists of deciding who you want to be. This involves choosing your identity, and proving it to yourself through small wins. These small wins can be acknowledged by rewarding yourself each time you resist distractions and prioritize your studies. Enjoy the process.

CHAPTER 3

PERSONALIZED LEARNING STYLES

The second component of neurohacking the learning cycle is personalize. What do we mean by personalize? On a biological level, personalize refers to the fact that we are all unique beings with different DNA and a blend of nature and nurture experiences. While our DNA provides a foundation, our early life experiences shape which genes become activated or deactivated. Even twins who share similar DNA have their individual experiences that influence their gene expression. The interplay between nature and nurture forms the essence of who we are.

The brain is astonishingly dynamic, especially during early development. At a young age, the brain starts with a basic set of neural connections, and with each experience the child develops new pathways and circuits. The exciting part is that every experience, even later in life, continues to reshape the brain and influence the DNA. There are two scientific phenomena which are occurring in this process: they are called neuroplasticity and epigenetics. Neuroplasticity is the brain's ability to rewire itself at any age. Epigenetics describes how every activity in our environment—our diet, exercise, and even meditation—can switch genes on or off. Regardless of the genes we inherit, our brain can be improved through the dynamics of neuroplasticity and epigenetics. We all have the power to change and rewire our brain. This ability is one of our greatest superpowers.

Learning how to practice Transcendental Meditation is an excellent starting point for this transformation. Each experience of transcending causes the neural pathways in your brain to undergo change. EEG scans of meditators reveal increased coherence and integration, with different parts of the brain connecting to each other more effectively. This enhanced connectivity aids in learning and also impacts emotions and, in fact, every aspect of life. Epigenetic research also shows that with the practice of meditation you are also changing gene expression, modifying which genes are turned on and off.

By making transcending a regular practice, something you do twice a day without conscious effort, you reinforce integration within your brain. Meditation becomes a powerful habit and a formula for success. TM is a technique that is available for everyone. It is taught personally to each individual. However, it is also something any person can do no matter what their background, education, and cultural or religious upbringing.

There are many aspects of the world that are being personalized for good or bad. In the field of health, a new field called personalized medicine has emerged in which your DNA is analyzed and then you are given drugs which best fit your specific genetic profile. In the area of social media, companies are constantly gathering data to personalize your advertisements and content whether you like it or not.

Our focus is on how we can improve your learning ability. Each of us has different preferences and approaches to learning. It's important to recognize and embrace these differences. Unfortunately, traditional learning systems often overlook the concept of diverse learning styles.

Learning Styles

During my early years, I (Carol) didn't consider myself particularly smart. While I excelled in language, math, and science, geography and history were a challenge for me. Even now, I still feel inadequate in geography. Interestingly, I realize that my perception of being "bad" at geography is tied to the identity I had assumed. I still need to work on letting go of that identity. As I grew older and began teaching adults, I discovered the existence of distinct learning styles. It dawned on me that I was never unintelligent; rather, the teaching methods used for history and geography didn't align with my preferred learning style.

For instance, those courses at my school primarily relied on lectures, which didn't suit my visual learning style. As a reader, I absorb information more effectively through visual aids and text. Consequently, I struggled to grasp the content presented through auditory lectures. This misconception haunted me for years, making me believe I was not a bright student. However, when I started teaching adults my perspective changed.

When I was teaching a class with 30 or 40 students, gathered in front of their computers to learn computer engineering, I observed an intriguing pattern. While introducing myself and the course, I noticed distinct behaviors among the students. Some individuals were visually inclined and looking at their computer screens or books, while others were actively listening. It's possible that some of you reading this right now identify as visual learners. On the other hand, some of you are auditory learners.

This initial observation provided valuable insight into each student's preferred learning style and allowed me to anticipate which sections of the course might pose challenges for different individuals. For instance, when it came to practical labs that required reading step-by-step instructions, auditory learners often encountered difficulties, while visual learners thrived. It was fascinating to witness these differences.

Recognizing that we all have distinct learning styles, we will guide you to identify your own preferred learning style. By understanding how you learn best, you can tailor your learning plan to suit your needs.

Let me share another personal story that illustrates this. When I began my master's degree at Maharishi International University, I watched a recorded lecture where doctors who were sitting in a long row of chairs introduced themselves one by one. Being enthusiastic about starting my degree, I eagerly watched the video. However, my focus quickly shifted to noticing that all the doctors were wearing tan suits. I started wondering if they were meant to wear tan suits and pondered the time of year that the video had been recorded. Lost in these thoughts, I completely missed the audio portion of the lecture, and I couldn't recall who each person was. As you now know, this is because I am more of a visual learner. To support my individual learning style, even when watching TV, I turn on closed captions since reading the text helps me stay engaged with the auditory content.

On the other hand, my husband, who is an auditory learner, shared a different experience. Early in our marriage, he mentioned that reading didn't captivate him, and he didn't feel that he was very skilled at it. I found this quite perplexing, since I cherished books. However, during our car rides to visit my mother, we started listening to audiobooks. One day, my husband surprised me by recalling specific details from the book, mentioning the chapter and when we heard it. It dawned on me that he is an auditory learner, and later, after taking an online test, he discovered that he is dyslexic. This realization shattered his belief that he wasn't smart or adept at book learning. In fact, he excels in auditory learning, and now we often get two copies of a book, a printed copy for me to read and an audiobook for him to listen to.

There are also individuals who are kinesthetic learners; they absorb information through physical movement and hands-on experiences. For instance, if you've ever received directions while driving and struggled to recall them later when alone, it's because kinesthetic learners benefit from actively doing tasks. They may consult maps, follow directions, and physically turn right or left, to solidify their understanding. If you identify as a kinesthetic learner, you can enhance your learning process by using colored pencils to take notes, incorporating tabs and sticky notes, or engaging in activities that involve physical contact. These strategies will contribute to a more effective learning experience.

Remember, some of us learn quickly, while others require more time. Each of us is unique, and the key to becoming the best student lies in understanding each individual's learning styles. Visual learners excel at absorbing knowledge from books and visual cues, while audio learners gravitate toward audio materials like lectures and audiobooks. Audio learners can also benefit from reading aloud sentences in textbooks, since this activity engages their ears as well. Lastly, kinesthetic learners can enhance their learning by incorporating physical movement and hands-on activities, such as cooking or engaging in tasks that involve touch. By recognizing and embracing our unique learning styles, we can optimize our learning potential and become the best version of ourselves as students.

Personalized Toolkit

Throughout this chapter, we have emphasized the importance of personalization in learning and highlighted reading as a fundamental tool for improving life and acquiring knowledge. While reading is a universal skill, it is taught to each of us individually rather than as a group. Once we have mastered reading, it becomes a lifelong asset that continuously reshapes our brain. The result? Reading grants us greater internal stability and enhances our ability to adapt to external circumstances—an especially valuable benefit.

We can explore a variety of other tools that will be discussed in subsequent lessons. These tools encompass practices like yoga, Ayurveda, exercise, diet, sleep, and various learning techniques. These are the components of a personalized toolkit that you can acquire, tailoring it to your specific needs and preferences. By identifying what works best for you—it might be yoga, a particular diet, exercise schedule, or other practices—you can create a daily routine that revolves around your individual strengths and needs. Our primary focus is to equip you with these tools, which will facilitate your personal learning process.

As we progress, we will explore a range of additional tools to enhance our learning experience. These tools can be customized to suit our needs, allowing us to build a personalized daily routine. By acquiring and implementing these tools, we can optimize our learning journey.

We recommend that you take the following assessment to help determine your own individualized learning style—whether you are more visual, auditory, or kinesthetic. This awareness is tremendously valuable. Once I discovered my preference for visual learning during my master's degree, I started transcribing videos to have the words on paper, which significantly enhanced my learning. Similarly, upon realizing my husband's inclination toward auditory learning, we now automatically obtain both printed and audio books, aligning with his preferred learning style. It's worth noting that you can embrace multiple learning styles simultaneously. Even though I lean more toward visual learning, I strive to become a better listener, so I often read aloud to engage both my auditory and visual senses when reading a book.

Once you have completed this assessment and identified your primary learning style, you will have the opportunity to tailor and adapt your study habits throughout the course. This assessment serves as a foundation for understanding yourself as a learner and empowers you to make intentional adjustments that cater to your specific needs.

What Type of Learner are You?

1. When exploring a new location, how do you navigate your way?
   a) Seek out a visual map or directory that provides an overview of the surroundings and points of interest.
   b) Approach someone for guidance and ask for directions.
   c) Begin wandering and exploring until you stumble upon what you're seeking.

2. What do you find to be the most disruptive while attempting to study?
   a) Individuals visually passing by your vicinity.
   b) Noises of high volume.
   c) An uneasy or uncomfortable chair.

3. How do you like to unwind and relax?

a) Engage in reading.

b) Listen to music.

c) Exercise through engaging activities like walking, running, or playing sports.

4. What tends to be your typical response when experiencing anger?

a) Donning a visual expression that conveys anger or frustration.

b) Raising your voice or shouting.

c) Forcefully shutting doors or causing them to slam shut.

5. What type of book would you prefer to read for enjoyment?

a) A book filled with captivating textual content.

b) A book abundant with illustrations or images.

c) A book featuring word searches or crossword puzzles.

6. How do you typically approach problem-solving or decision-making?

a) By visualizing the potential outcomes and weighing the pros and cons.

b) By discussing the options and considering different viewpoints.

c) By physically trying out different approaches or experimenting to find a solution.

7. What is your preferred method for remembering a friend's phone number?

a) Visualize the numbers as you would visually dial them on a phone keypad.

   b) Repeatedly vocalize the number out loud.

   c) Jot it down or save it in your phone's contact list.

8. How do you prefer to learn a new skill or activity?

   a) By watching videos or demonstrations.

   b) By listening to instructions or explanations.

   c) By physically engaging in the activity and practicing hands-on.

9. After attending a party, what aspect would you most likely retain in your memory the following day?

   a) The visually memorable people who were present.

   b) The music that was playing during the party.

   c) The appealing food that you consumed.

10. What type of classroom environment do you find most conducive to your learning?

   a) A visually organized and aesthetically pleasing space.

   b) An environment with minimal noise or distractions.

   c) A classroom that allows for physical movement and hands-on learning opportunities.

11. While waiting in line at the grocery store, what would you typically do?

   a) Engage in visually observing the products displayed on nearby racks.

   b) Strike up a conversation with the individual standing next to you in line.

   c) Display restlessness or exhibit back-and-forth movements.

12. What tends to be the most distracting factor while in a classroom?

  a) Excessive brightness or dimness of the lights.

  b) Noises emanating from the hallway or outside the building, such as traffic or lawn mowing.

  c) Uncomfortably hot or cold temperature in the room.

13. What type of presentation or learning material captures your attention the most?

  a) Visual presentations with images, charts, or graphs.

  b) Auditory presentations with engaging speakers or interactive discussions.

  c) Hands-on demonstrations or activities that involve movement and physical interaction.

14. How do you typically retain information in your memory?

  a) By visualizing images or diagrams related to the information.

  b) By repeating or vocalizing the information to yourself.

  c) By physically writing or actively engaging with the information.

15. What actions do you usually engage in when feeling joyful?

  a) Displaying a broad visual smile that stretches from ear to ear.

  b) Engaging in lively and extensive conversations.

  c) Exhibiting exuberant behavior or hyperactivity.

16. What is the most effective method for you to prepare for an examination?

  a) Engage in visually reading the book or your notes

while also reviewing visual aids like pictures or charts.

b) Utilize a question-and-answer approach, where someone quizzes you, and you respond verbally.

c) Create index cards that can be used for review purposes

17. When encountering uncertainty spelling a word, what is your typical course of action?

a) Jot it down to visually assess its correctness.

b) Pronounce it aloud to gauge its auditory accuracy.

c) Employ finger spelling by tracing the letters in the air.

18. If you were to win a game, which prize would you choose from these three options?

a) A visually appealing poster to adorn your wall.

b) A music CD or a downloadable mp3.

c) A game or a sports-related item like a football or soccer ball.

19. What aspect about new individuals you meet is most likely to stick in your memory?

a) Remembering their face but not their name.

b) Recalling their name but not their face.

c) Retaining engaging information about the conversations you had with them.

20. Which of these options would you rather attend with a group of friends?

a) Watching a movie together.

b) Attending a concert.

    c) Visiting an amusement park.

21. Among these three subjects, which class do you prefer the most?

    a) Art class

    b) Music class

    c) Gym class

22. When a song plays on the radio, what is your typical response?

    a) Imagine the corresponding music video in your mind.

    b) Sing or hum along with the music.

    c) Start dancing or tapping your foot in rhythm.

23. When providing directions to your house, what would you most likely say to someone?

    a) Offer a detailed description of the building and notable landmarks they will encounter along the way.

    b) Provide the names of roads or streets they will traverse.

    c) Suggest, "Follow me—it will be easier if I personally show you how to get there."

How to Score the Quiz

Assign one point to each answer choice based on the learning style it represents:

- For "a)" answers indicating a visual learning style,

assign 1 point.

- For "b)" answers indicating an auditory learning style, assign 1 point.

- For "c)" answers indicating a kinesthetic learning style, assign 1 point.

Add up the points associated with each letter.

Visual Learner

If you have the highest points in the "a" answer (visual learning style), then your dominant learning style is visual.

If you possess a visual learning style, you acquire knowledge through reading and visual representations. Your understanding and retention of information are primarily influenced by sight. You have the ability to create mental images of what you are learning, and visual methods are most effective for your learning process. Observing and seeing the material is crucial to your comprehension.

As a visual learner, you typically exhibit tidiness and cleanliness. When trying to visualize or recall something, you often close your eyes, and if you find yourself bored, you seek something visually stimulating to focus on. Spoken instructions may pose challenges for you, and you may be easily distracted by sounds. You are drawn to color and appreciate language that evokes vivid imagery, such as stories.

Auditory Learner

If you have the highest points in the "b" answers (auditory learning style), then your dominant learning style is auditory.

As an auditory learner, you have a preference for learning through hearing and listening. You comprehend and retain information that you have heard. You rely on the sound of information to store it in your memory, and you find it easier to understand instructions when they are spoken rather than written. Reading aloud is a beneficial learning method for you because you need to hear or speak the information to grasp it.

If you are an auditory learner, you may engage in humming or talking to yourself or others when you feel bored. Despite appearances, you often pay attention to and comprehend everything that is being said.

Kinesthetic Learner

If you have the highest points in the "c" answers (kinesthetic learning style), then your dominant learning style is kinesthetic.

If you are a kinesthetic or tactile learner, you acquire knowledge through touch and physical involvement. You understand and remember information by engaging in physical movement. As a hands-on learner, you prefer to touch, manipulate, build, or draw to reinforce your learning. Activities involving physical movement enhance your learning experience, and you may struggle with sitting still for extended periods. You tend to use gestures and hand movements while speaking, and you often find reasons to engage in physical activity when you feel bored. You might possess good coordination skills and athletic abilities. Remembering actions or physical experiences comes naturally to you, while recalling visual or auditory information can be more challenging. Physical touch is an important aspect of your communication style, and you appreciate supportive gestures such as a pat on the back.

The scoring instructions provided above assume a single learning style dominance based on the highest point value but it is not uncommon for individuals to find themselves to be a combination of 2 or more learning styles. The key is to understand your learning style and then use that knowledge to enhance your learning abilities.

CHAPTER 4

PERSONALIZE WITH AYURVEDA

We are now going to personalized neurohacking through the ancient science of Ayurveda. What exactly is Ayurveda? Ayurveda is an ancient science of life that dates back 5000 years. The term "Ayu" means life, and "Veda" means science. These profound teachings have stood the test of time because they remain relevant and valuable to this day. While the knowledge originated thousands of years ago, its principles are highly applicable in our modern lives. Maharishi Mahesh Yogi, the founder of the Transcendental Meditation program, revived Ayurveda and brought back the understanding that consciousness is the foundation of everything. While Ayurveda has existed for a long time, the emphasis on consciousness was lost over time, with more focus being put on herbs and other aspects.

According to Ayurveda, everything in the universe is ultimately consciousness and manifesting from consciousness are the different forms of the five fundamental elements: space, air, fire, water, and earth. These elements form the basis of our being. Ayurveda further refines this understanding by identifying three basic doshas or underlying forces which govern our physiology.

These are called Vata, Pitta, and Kapha. Vata is a combination of air and space, Pitta is a blend of fire and water, and Kapha consists of earth and water elements. Each person is born with a different combination of these doshas. Identifying your predominant combination of doshas doesn't mean you walk around defining yourself solely by those elements. Instead, it signifies that you may resonate more with certain elements compared to others. For instance, I (Carol) am a blend of space and air, which means I have a light and dynamic aspect to my personality. Additionally, I possess fiery and watery traits, which give a great deal of energy. On the other hand, my husband is more grounded, representing an earth and water composition. Our different learning styles can be attributed to the unique elements that comprise our being.

The key point to understand here is that no Ayurvedic combination (Vata, Pitta, Kapha) is superior to any others. Whether you have a Pitta-Kapha constitution or any other combination, we are all wonderful in our own way. Each combination contributes to the whole and is equally important. Individuals are born with a specific combination, but it may change throughout their lives. It's similar to our DNA, which remains constant, yet different genes are expressed at different times in life. Even more important is the idea that certain behaviors can cause our doshas to become upset or imbalanced. We believe that understanding your Ayurvedic composition and how it becomes out of balance will enable you to improve your learning ability.

Vata Energy State Learners

In any classroom setting, you'll find a mix of quick and slow learners. Individuals with a predominantly Vata nature are usually the fastest at learning new concepts but they also have a tendency to forget quickly. They are often creative, imaginative, and full of new ideas. If you are a Vata learner, it is essential to establish enjoyable routines that nourish, please, and ground you. We will provide you with some surprisingly simple tips that will greatly support your learning and overall well-being.

Here are some practical suggestions for individuals with a Vata or V Energy State. Since you have a natural inclination for creativity, it's important to nurture and embrace your creative nature in the learning process. One way to do this is by using colored pens or pencils when taking notes. This simple act adds a fun and creative element, bringing your notes to life and enhancing your focus and attention.

Establishing a routine can also help you manage the constant movement of your body and mind. Set a specific time and place for studying to create a sense of structure and focus. This routine will support your learning process and help channel your energy effectively.

When it comes to your diet, opt for warm, cooked, and nourishing foods. Since Vata is a combination of space and air, it helps to eat foods that help ground you. Avoid consuming excessive amounts of dry foods like crackers and chips, as they can disrupt your body's balance. Adequate sleep is especially important for a

Vata, so make sure you prioritize getting enough rest.

As a part Vata person myself, (Carol) I find that I study best in the morning when my mind is rested and clear. Experiment with different times of the day to identify when your brain is most coherent and receptive to absorbing information. For me, reading something in the morning sets a positive tone for the day and enhances my learning experience.

Pitta Energy State Learners

What exactly is the nature of a Pitta or P Energy State individual? They are goal-oriented, focused, and are good at making positive changes in their life. Most habit books are written by Pitta people for Pitta people, which can leave other types feeling left out. Pitta individuals thrive by taking action. They are great at making lists and prioritizing tasks. In a group setting, you'll find them swiftly creating their to-do lists, and taking charge of the whole meeting.

Pitta individuals possess clarity and strong determination. They are purposeful and driven, often displaying a competitive nature. Understanding this aspect of their personality is key.

There is a wealth of advice available for Pitta individuals regarding diet, sleep, and other aspects. The most important tip for Pitta individuals to stay in balance is to not miss a meal. This can result in them becoming "hangry." Pitta individuals are composed of fire and water elements, so it is also important for them to not get overheated and to stay hydrated. Consuming overly spicy foods, can cause hyperacidity. Because Pittas are so energetic, they can overdo it at any time and not get enough sleep. Sleep is a fundamental requirement for everyone, as it plays a vital role in our overall well-being and productivity.

Pitta individuals often strive for perfection. It's important for them to use mistakes as valuable learning opportunities. These can provide deeper insights and enhance your understanding. I (Carol) am part Pitta and can personally attest that many of my learnings stem from past mistakes.

Focus on enjoying the learning process for the sake of knowledge acquisition, rather than solely striving for perfect grades. Recognize that at the end of your degree, when you receive your diploma, you'll be among peers who have also achieved the same milestone. Nobody in the crowd will be able to identify whether someone obtained their degree with all Bs or all As. The ultimate goal is obtaining the degree itself.

If you create a new study habit, such as establishing a specific time to do your homework, align this new habit with a long-term goal such as continuously improving your learning ability. Embrace your journey of learning, become addicted to the process of acquiring knowledge, and find joy in teaching others.

Kapha Energy State Learners

Kapha or K Energy State individuals are steady and consistent.

They prefer fixed routines and have a methodical and thorough approach to learning. Although it may take them a bit longer to fully grasp a new concept, once they've learned something, it remains ingrained in their memory.

How can you help a Kapha person to learn? When presenting them with a new study habit, give them enough time to fully think about it and realize its value in their lives. Don't hurry them, be patient. Let them think about it. They enjoy their routines, and their first reaction is to resist change. However, if the new ideas are presented over time and they can talk about it with a friend the change is easier for them. Once they adopt the new program, they are good at consistently sticking with it. Having a buddy or a supportive group can make a significant difference for a Kapha person since they are naturally social, friendly, and warm. The presence of friends provides the necessary motivation and support for them to embrace new habits effectively.

Let's explore some Ayurvedic suggestions for how to keep a Kapha or K Energy State person in balance. These individuals benefit from keeping their bodies and minds active. Taking a refreshing morning walk or engaging in any form of exercise can help invigorate their calm and grounded nature.

When it comes to their diet, Kaphas tend to have a slower digestion, so it helps if they consume lighter meals. Heavy and sweet foods tend to weigh them down, making them feel sluggish and lethargic. By opting for smaller meals with invigorating spices like ginger, they can maintain a more optimal digestive state.

Staying engaged with their studies helps Kapha individuals.

They also do better when together with other students since by nature they are social beings. Forming study groups is highly recommended. Working with others who possess different energies can be mutually beneficial, so each student can complement and support each other's learning styles.

Kaphas have a natural inclination toward sleep and can oversleep or have a hard time getting up in the morning. Extra sleep is good for them. It just has to be included in their schedule.

We have included a brief quiz at the end of this chapter so that you can assess your own Energy State. It is not as precise as an in-person analysis from an Ayurvedic expert, but it will give you a general idea. There is an intriguing and rare energy type in which all three scores are similar. In Ayurveda, this is known as a "tri dosha" type, referring to an equal combination of Vata, Pitta, and Kapha. It's an interesting and unique person who has an equal balance of all three energy states.

It's important to emphasize that each Energy State type has its own unique attributes, and understanding your Energy State type allows you to learn more about yourself, how you learn, and how you study. By utilizing this knowledge, you can surpass your own expectations and achieve greater success.

Even as children there are noticeable differences. Personally, during my two pregnancies, I (Carol) could sense the contrast between my two children. The older one was always quiet, making me worry about his lack of movement in my womb, while the younger one was constantly active, resembling a boxer. It's fascinating how these traits are expressed early on. Remember, there is no disadvantage or advantage in being any specific type. The key is to know your type and utilize that knowledge to tailor your learning style for your own benefit. That's what you'll gain from this assessment.

It's fascinating to note that there is a scientific basis to the Ayurvedic Energy States. Understanding who you are allows you to better personalize, enabling you to optimize your life and maintain a better balance. The central focus here is on utilizing this knowledge to enhance your well-being and improve your learning ability.

Energy State Quiz

V Energy State	*Strongly Disagree / Strongly Agree*				
1. Light sleeper, difficulty falling asleep	[1]	[2]	[3]	[4]	[5]
2. Irregular appetite	[1]	[2]	[3]	[4]	[5]
3. Learns quickly but forgets quickly	[1]	[2]	[3]	[4]	[5]
4. Easily becomes overstimulated	[1]	[2]	[3]	[4]	[5]
5. Does not tolerate cold weather very well	[1]	[2]	[3]	[4]	[5]
6. A sprinter rather than a marathoner	[1]	[2]	[3]	[4]	[5]
7. Speech is energetic, with frequent changes in topic	[1]	[2]	[3]	[4]	[5]
8. Anxious and worried when under stress	[1]	[2]	[3]	[4]	[5]
V Score	*(Total your responses)*				

P Energy State	Strongly Disagree / Strongly Agree				
1. Easily becomes overheated	[1]	[2]	[3]	[4]	[5]
2. Strong reaction when challenged	[1]	[2]	[3]	[4]	[5]
3. Uncomfortable when meals are delayed	[1]	[2]	[3]	[4]	[5]
4. Good at physical activity	[1]	[2]	[3]	[4]	[5]
5. Strong appetite	[1]	[2]	[3]	[4]	[5]
6. Good sleeper but may not need as much sleep as others	[1]	[2]	[3]	[4]	[5]
7. Clear and precise speech	[1]	[2]	[3]	[4]	[5]
8. Becomes irritable and/or angry under stress	[1]	[2]	[3]	[4]	[5]
P Score	(Total your responses)				

K ENERGY STATE	STRONGLY DISAGREE / STRONGLY AGREE				
1. Slow eater	[1]	[2]	[3]	[4]	[5]
2. Falls asleep easily but wakes up slowly	[1]	[2]	[3]	[4]	[5]
3. Steady, stable temperament	[1]	[2]	[3]	[4]	[5]
4. Doesn't mind waiting to eat	[1]	[2]	[3]	[4]	[5]
5. Slow to learn but rarely forgets	[1]	[2]	[3]	[4]	[5]
6. Good physical strength and stamina	[1]	[2]	[3]	[4]	[5]
7. Speech may be slow and thoughtful	[1]	[2]	[3]	[4]	[5]
8. Possessive and stubborn under stress	[1]	[2]	[3]	[4]	[5]
K SCORE	(TOTAL YOUR RESPONSES)				

Compare all three scores. Whichever total is higher, V, P, or K, is your primary Energy State. It is common to have two high scores and one lower score. This shows that you are a combination of two main Energy States, with a minor influence from the third. In some cases, you may have three similar scores. This is somewhat rare and indicates that you are a Tri-Energy State. You may also find that your score highlights only one Energy State. This means that every aspect of your life is strongly influenced by this Energy State.

CHAPTER 5

CREATING A NEUROHACK MAP AND PLAN

We have already covered Motivate and Personalize, now it's time to delve into Experiment. Experimenting plays a vital role in learning. To assist you in this process we'll give you a formula for effortlessly cultivating new habits.

Step 1

Create a Neurohack Map—Begin by placing your main intention or desire for the neurohack in the center of a blank piece of paper or your computer screen. This could be something like "Finish my homework on time" or "Be regular in my meditation."

Step 2

Expand Your Neurohack Map—Around the central idea, imagine spokes radiating from the hub of a wheel. List specific action steps that you believe will help you achieve the desired change, breaking down the central idea into smaller, concrete steps. For instance, "setting a designated time for homework" or "participating in online group meditation".

Step 3

Develop Your Neurohack Plan—Now it's time to create your plan based on the Neurohack Map. Prioritize your list of action steps and choose the main habit that will be the focus of your initial experiment. For example, designate a specific study or meditation time.

Step 4

Implement Your Neurohack Plan—Select a cue or prompt that will remind you to perform your chosen habit. This could involve setting a phone reminder for your designated study or meditation time.

Step 5

Measure Your Success—Determine how you will measure your progress and success in adopting the new habit. Consider creating a calendar where you can mark your successful completion of the habit. Once this is done, reward yourself. You can break it down into rewards for the first week, first month, or even the first year.

Now let's look at a couple of examples of Neurohack Maps and Plans.

Brianna

Brianna is an individual with a predominant V Energy State. She is a tall, thin blonde woman in her mid-thirties and she is generally healthy. However, she tends to catch colds and the flu easily, often being the first among her friends to fall ill. She dislikes the cold and prefers warmth. Brianna works as a graphic designer in Florida.

Now, let's delve into Brianna's neurohack map, focusing first on her main desire in the center. Brianna wants to be a better student by submitting her homework on time. From the center of the map, three items extend outward like spokes on a bicycle wheel. These represent three action items that Brianna thinks will assist her in achieving her neurohack.

The first action item is practicing regular Transcendental Meditation. Brianna believes that TM can bring her more mental clarity and focus to her somewhat scattered personality. The second action item is reviewing assignments in advance. Brianna believes that by examining assignments early on, she can better organize her efforts to complete weekly goals. The third action item is creating a dedicated homework time. Brianna feels that setting aside specific time solely for homework will help her meet deadlines.

Brianna now prioritizes her three new actions and determines that reviewing assignments at the beginning of the week is crucial for establishing structure and organization in her workflow. To make this neurohack easier to implement, Brianna establishes a routine centered around reviewing her assignments. She decides to make this process a part of her morning ritual, immediately after enjoying her cup of tea. This allows her to calmly assess the tasks at hand and estimate the time required to complete them. By not reviewing assignments in the evening before bed, Brianna avoids the potential restlessness caused by an overly active mind, particularly since V Energy State people often face challenges with sleep.

Next, Brianna selects a neurohack buddy to help her track her progress. This buddy will ask her every week whether she reviewed her upcoming assignments and allocated dedicated study time to complete them. Brianna understands the importance of having someone else involved to keep her grounded and accountable.

As a reward for successfully reviewing her assignments on time for a month, Brianna plans to treat herself to a 10 milliliter bottle of lavender or rose organic essential oil. This serves as a tangible reward for her effort, in addition to the satisfaction she gains knowing that she consistently planned ahead each week.

BRIANNA'S – NEUROHACK MAP & PLAN

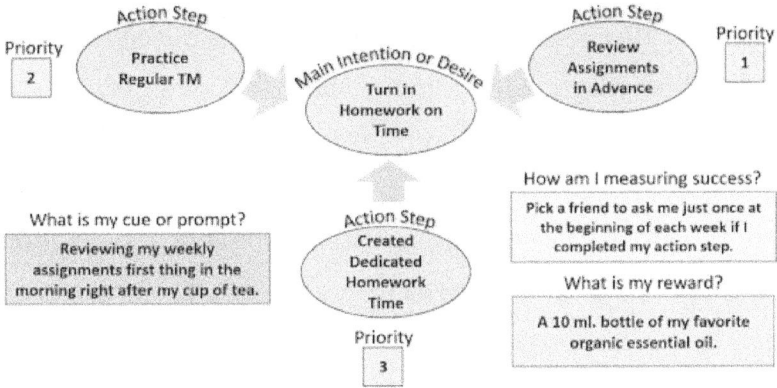

Action Step

Priority
2

Practice
Regular TM

Main Intention or Desire

Turn in
Homework on
Time

Action Step

Review
Assignments
in Advance

Priority
1

What is my cue or prompt?

Reviewing my weekly
assignments first thing in the
morning right after my cup of tea.

Action Step

Created
Dedicated
Homework
Time

Priority
3

How am I measuring success?

Pick a friend to ask me just once at
the beginning of each week if I
completed my action step.

What is my reward?

A 10 ml. bottle of my favorite
organic essential oil.

Lauren

Lauren, is a K energy type. She has a somewhat stocky build, mysterious brown eyes with long and lovely eyelashes, and thick dark hair. Lauren is a skilled gourmet cook and has successfully managed a cooking specialty shop for several years. She is beloved by her employees. However, when she returns home from work, she prefers to relax in front of the TV. This often leads to lethargy and boredom, preventing her from taking the actions necessary to complete her degree. As mentioned earlier, the K energy type requires enthusiasm and drive, which can be lacking in Lauren's case. She realizes she needs additional motivation to stay engaged during her studies. Let's examine Lauren's Neurohack Map.

Lauren's primary goal is to stay motivated, which is reflected in the center of her map. Surrounding this central idea, like spokes on a wheel, are the actions or experiments she believes will help her achieve this goal. One action is to associate studying with a delightful beverage. For example, she could designate chai tea as her studying treat, allowing herself to indulge only when she is doing her homework. Another idea is to find a study buddy. This can help balance her own personality and bring in a diverse perspective, leading to remarkable outcomes. One final idea is to pick a particular study time each day which would work for her, since she loves to have a fixed schedule. These are the three actions Lauren has identified.

Lauren prioritizes her actions steps. She decides to focus on finding a neurohack buddy who can keep her motivated and accountable during her studies. This buddy will help prevent boredom and lethargy, particularly if they are a complementary type such as a P or V Energy State individual. Lauren plans to set reminders (her prompt) on her phone to ensure she doesn't miss any study sessions with her neurohack buddy, addressing her tendency to become engrossed in enjoyable activities and neglect commitments.

As for measuring success, she intends to ask a trusted friend to call every evening and inquire about her dedication to her neurohack plan and study sessions. This external accountability will help keep her on track. For a reward, Lauren, who is friendly and sociable, decides to celebrate her achievements at the end of week one by going out to lunch with friends. This will provide a sense of satisfaction and further motivate her.

LAUREN'S – NEUROHACK MAP & PLAN

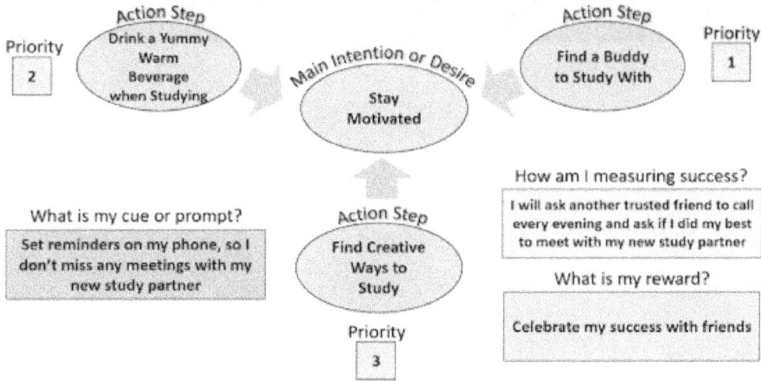

Action Step

Priority
2

Drink a Yummy Warm Beverage when Studying

Main Intention or Desire

Stay Motivated

Action Step

Find a Buddy to Study With

Priority
1

How am I measuring success?

I will ask another trusted friend to call every evening and ask if I did my best to meet with my new study partner

What is my cue or prompt?

Set reminders on my phone, so I don't miss any meetings with my new study partner

Action Step

Find Creative Ways to Study

Priority
3

What is my reward?

Celebrate my success with friends

Below is a graphic so you can make your own neurohack map and plan. In the center, enter your main intention or desire for the neurohack. Focus on an area where you feel you need assistance, preferably related to your studies. However, it can pertain to any aspect of your life that requires improvement. Around this central circle, in the three ovals, list three action steps that you believe will help you achieve the central goal. After listing these steps, in the boxes outside the ovals, prioritize them based on their ease of implementation. Choose the one you can tackle first, as you only need one for your neurohack plan. In the light box on the right, describe your cue or prompt, which will remind you to maintain the chosen action step. Determine how you will measure your success and decide on a reward for yourself. Enjoy the process.

NEUROHACK MAP & PLAN

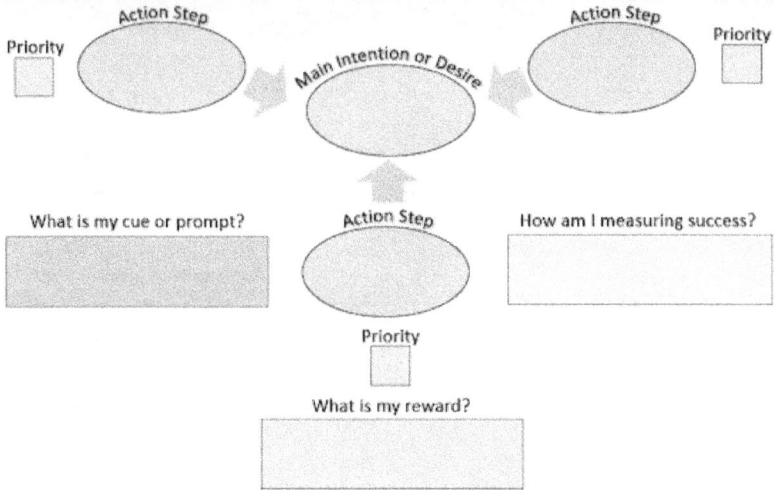

Action Step

Priority

Main Intention or Desire

Action Step

Priority

What is my cue or prompt?

Action Step

How am I measuring success?

Priority

What is my reward?

CHAPTER 6

LIFESTYLE HABITS FOR BETTER LEARNING

How can you improve your ability to adopt new study habits? One thing to realize is that there are many factors which influence your motivation and therefore your ability to experiment successfully. Sometimes you need to start with some simple neurohacks and habits which will help improve your focus and energy level.

The Transcendental Meditation program, for example, is a simple neurohack. We could also call it a Super Habit since it improves your clarity, concentration, and many other aspects which are relevant to studying. Other simple neurohacks include changes in diet, exercise, and sleep. It is hard to study if your stomach is upset, or you are tired.

Ayurveda provides personalized knowledge for each of these areas that has been successfully applied over many thousands of years. When the techniques of Ayurveda are combined with the latest knowledge of modern health, we can make significant improvements in our diet, exercise, sleep, and stress management. These changes all help us to increase our energy level and ability to focus on our studies. Let's consider each of these areas briefly.

Diet

Diet and digestion play a significant role in learning. If your gut is upset, it is hard to study. We now know that our gut affects every part of our body. The latest research has revealed the importance of our microbiome, which is the friendly bacteria and other microorganisms that live in our gut. The gut is directly connected to the brain and therefore has a big impact on our mental health and learning ability. Researchers have identified the gut-brain axis which shows that the gut is connected to the nervous system, endocrine system, and immune system. Our gut microbiome acts as a specialized organ within us and has a profound impact on our overall well-being. For instance, studies have shown that probiotics can help individuals cope with stress.

What we eat directly affects our gut microbiome, which in turn influences every part of our body, particularly our energy levels and ability to focus. Many people talk about "brain fog," which often is caused by our poor diet and digestion. This understanding aligns with the age-old saying, "You are what you eat." Currently, people consume unhealthy fast food due to the constraints of time and cost. Often these processed foods are loaded with additives, salt, and sugar, which create a craving for more. Unfortunately, this trend has led to a rise in issues like irritable bowel syndrome, one of the most common digestive problems. There is a gut crisis.

Diet and digestion hold immense importance in Ayurveda and there are many positive simple habits that can improve the health of our digestive tract. There are general recommendations for everyone to follow, and more importantly there are personalized recommendations for each Energy State.

The Vata or V Energy State individuals have a variable appetite, sometimes feeling hungry and other times not. Their digestive power also fluctuates, with some foods being digested quickly while others take longer. It benefits them to have multiple small and nutritious meals throughout the day to maintain a steady supply of nutrients. Creating a calm and stress-free environment for meals is incredibly important for them. It is advised not to eat while standing up or in a car. Instead, they should treat each meal as a special moment, sitting down and savoring the experience. This is important for their body to digest food properly. When out of balance, Vata individuals may experience symptoms like constipation, indigestion, and gas. Encountering any of these symptoms suggests that your eating habits might not have been optimal, leading to these issues.

Pitta or P Energy State individuals generally have strong digestion, allowing them to eat a wide variety of food. This is especially true of a young Pitta individual who can indulge in ice cream and pizza late at night and still have a good night's sleep. One critical factor with Pitta digestion is the need to eat on time. The concept of "hangry" perfectly fits a P Energy State individual who can get irritable and even angry when they miss a meal.

Ayurveda recommends for everyone to eat their main meal at lunch. This is the meal a P Energy State person should not miss. The fiery nature of Pitta can result in acid reflux and indigestion when they consume excessively hot spicy foods or when their body is out of balance.

The Kapha or K Energy State individual has a steady and slower digestive system. They can miss a meal and not be upset. Kaphas have a genuine love for food. However, due to their slower metabolism they are prone to gaining weight. Excessive sweets and other heavy foods can make them feel lethargic. It is advisable for Kaphas to opt for lighter food choices.

There are two books coauthored by Dr. Wallace that contain valuable information about these subjects. The first book, *Gut Crisis,* focuses on the gut microbiome and how you can keep it in balance. The second book, *The Rest and Repair Diet*, presents a step-by-step diet plan, suitable for both vegetarians and meat eaters, designed to improve overall health. While weight loss is a side benefit, the primary goal of the rest and repair diet is to restore and rejuvenate your diet and digestion to their optimal state. It contains numerous recipes and serves as a valuable tool for resting and repairing your digestive system.

Exercise

Another powerful supportive habit that can improve your learning ability and overall health is exercise, especially yoga asanas. Nowadays, exercise is highly recommended by doctors and experts alike, and for good reason. Engaging in physical activity, even something as simple as taking a walk, offers numerous benefits for both mental and physical health. It's crucial to make time for regular exercise as part of your learning journey.

Yoga is good for all Energy State types and has been extensively studied and proven to provide a wide range of benefits to enhance your overall well-being. The practice of Maharishi Yoga Asana is an ideal daily routine for the body and mind. It also includes a breathing exercise (pranayama practice) which is good for both your health and learning ability.

For a Vata or V Energy State person the best types of exercise are dynamic agile activities that don't strain or overtire them. Moderate workouts are recommended. Activities such as dancing, paddleboarding, and yoga are often enjoyed by Vata types.

Pitta Energy State individuals need lots of exercise and often excel in athletics due to their good stamina and strength. They have a competitive nature and thrive in organized sports, especially team sports, which provide a fantastic outlet for their abundant energy. However, considering their fiery nature, it's essential for Pitta individuals to avoid overheating. Excessive exposure to the sun can lead to overheating, which is why engaging in active water sports becomes an ideal choice. Activities like swimming, surfing, and parasailing help keep the Pitta type cool and refreshed. Even when playing team sports, taking a dip in the pool or a lake afterward can significantly lower their body temperature and make a noticeable difference.

When discussing the Pitta Energy State type, I (Carol) was reminded of a client I once had who frequently lost his temper while playing outdoor sports. He couldn't understand why he wasn't able to control his temper until his assessment revealed that he was a Pitta type. He was exercising in the middle of the day under the scorching sun. The additional heat was aggravating his temper during the game. He sought my help in finding a solution to balance his temper, and we primarily focused on adjusting his exercise time and diet. This simple change made a significant difference for him.

Kapha or K Energy State individuals typically excel in strength and endurance. Regular physical exercise is essential for them to avoid feeling sluggish and becoming overweight. It's crucial for Kapha types to get moving, and the easiest way to start is by taking a morning walk or engaging in activities like running, jogging, or energetic gym workouts. The key is to be active and avoid a sedentary lifestyle. Walking with friends, in particular, is a wonderful exercise option.

Sleep

Getting enough sleep is incredibly important for our overall well-being. Researchers continue to uncover the many essential functions that occur during sleep. One such function is the cleaning role of the glymphatic system (different from the lymphatic system), which works to eliminate toxins that accumulate in the brain throughout the day. Additionally, sleep plays a vital role in memory consolidation and other critical processes that are essential for our daily lives as well as for learning.

Numerous studies have been conducted on individuals who experience sleep problems such as those with insomnia or those who work night shifts. These studies consistently reveal that inadequate sleep leads to poor performance and various health issues. Therefore, the quality of our sleep is of utmost importance.

The factors influencing sleep quality differ for each individual based on their unique energy state. It is crucial for each person to be aware of these factors and take them into consideration when aiming for restful sleep.

Individuals with a Vata or V Energy State often struggle with falling asleep and are prone to experiencing insomnia. It is crucial for them to take extra precautions to avoid activities or stimuli that can disrupt their sleep. One key recommendation is to minimize exposure to stimulating devices such as computers and cell phones before bed. The artificial light emitted by these devices can interfere with the natural production of melatonin, a hormone that promotes sleep. Ideally, going to bed by 10 p.m. is considered the optimal time for sleep. Therefore, Vata types should refrain from using electronic digital devices after 8 pm to give themselves some stimulus-free transition time. It is advisable to keep these devices out of reach, turned off, or stored in a drawer.

To enhance the chances of having a restful night's sleep, Vata individuals can incorporate relaxing activities into their bedtime routine. Taking a soothing warm bath, listening to peaceful music, and using calming aromatherapy can aid in promoting relaxation. Personal preferences, such as using an Amazon Echo device to play nature sounds, can also contribute to a soothing sleep environment. Exploring various grounding strategies tailored to balance their dynamic Vata Energy State can help improve sleep quality for these individuals.

Pitta individuals typically require less sleep and fall asleep easily since sleep comes naturally and effortlessly. However, it is not uncommon for them to experience occasional awakenings during the night due to their abundant energy. It is essential for them to maintain balance and avoid eating overly spicy foods that may cause hyperacidity. By prioritizing overall balance and well-being, Pitta individuals can ensure that their sleep remains undisturbed.

Individuals with a Kapha Energy State have no trouble falling asleep due to their love for comfort. They find solace in climbing into bed and experiencing a hibernation-like sleep. However, waking up in the morning can be challenging for them, and they often require more time to prepare for the day. To counteract this, engaging in a morning walk is essential for Kapha types as it helps awaken their energy.

There are various strategies to assist Kapha individuals in waking up, including using alarm clocks that gradually illuminate the room with light. It's crucial for Kaphas to prioritize getting sufficient sleep by aiming to be in bed by 10 p.m. By doing so, they can easily rise at 6 a.m., while still ensuring they have enjoyed a blissful 8 hours of sleep. Conversely, staying up late, such as until midnight or 1 a.m., will result in them feeling tired and lethargic when the alarm goes off at 6 a.m., affecting their entire day. To maintain a vibrant and energized state, Kapha individuals should prioritize their sleep and incorporate morning movement into their routine.

Start Small

Throughout our discussion, we've explored various innovative neurohacks. To enhance your life, we want you to choose a specific intention or desire to help in your sleep habits. If you currently go to bed at midnight, aiming for 10:00 pm might be too drastic of a change. Instead, consider a smaller shift, like going to bed at 11:30 pm. This half-hour change will hardly be noticeable, yet it will bring you closer to neurohacking your life for improved health, happiness, and academic success. Once your goal is reached, you can adjust it again.

Use the graphic below and begin by placing your main intention or desire in the center of your map. For example, your main intention might be to go to bed at an earlier time. Then, identify three action steps that you believe will help you achieve your goal. In the boxes, prioritize these steps based on what you can implement right away to progress toward your main objective.

Next, determine the prompts or cues you'll use to support your desired action. To go to bed earlier, you might set an alarm on your phone an hour before your desired bedtime to initiate your wind-down routine. As for measuring success, consider marking a calendar each day you complete a neurohack that supports your sleep.

Additionally, think about the rewards you'll grant yourself for your efforts. Naturally, you'll feel the initial reward of improved well-being as the week progresses and you practice these neurohacks. However, consider a tangible reward, such as treating yourself to a $5 Amazon purchase or something within your budget that brings you joy. Be creative in selecting a reward that motivates you. Fill in the graphic below.

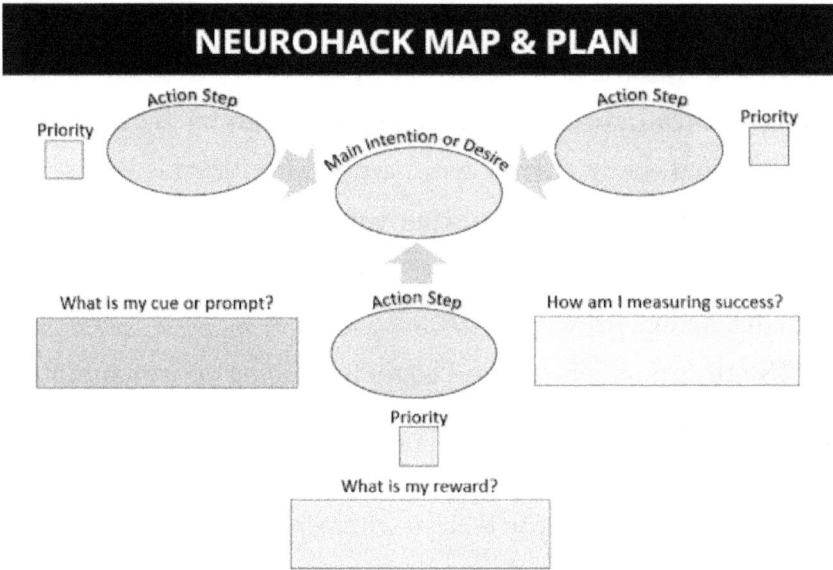

NEUROHACK MAP & PLAN

Action Step

Priority

Main Intention or Desire

Action Step

Priority

What is my cue or prompt?

Action Step

How am I measuring success?

Priority

What is my reward?

CHAPTER 7

NEUROHACKING WITH MORNING SUNLIGHT

Various health systems, including Ayurveda, have long recognized the significance of maintaining consistent biorhythms and routines for optimal health. Almost all forms of life, from bacteria to humans, possess an internal biological clock that operates on a roughly 24-hour circadian rhythm.

Jet lag occurs when individuals travel to a different time zone, disrupting their biological clock due to variations in sunlight, sunrise, and sunset. Perhaps you have even experienced it yourself or witnessed it in others. I (Carol) recall attending slumber parties when I was young. I would stay up way past my regular bedtime. The following day, I would often experience digestive discomfort. This was a result of disturbing my body's natural biorhythms and throwing my stomach bacteria out of balance. It is an example of how crucial it is to maintain our daily routines and biorhythms.

Synchronizing Biological Clocks

Morning sunlight is an easily accessible and enjoyable

neurohack. Sunlight consists of visible light, often referred to as white light, since it contains all the colors of the rainbow. Have you ever wondered why the sky appears blue? It's because the blue wavelengths of light, being short in size, scatter when they encounter air molecules in the atmosphere. We typically observe this blue sky phenomenon around noon.

When light enters the eye, it interacts with various pigments, allowing us to perceive visual information. These pigments are found in cells in the back of the eye in the retina. The rod cells contain the pigment rhodopsin which is good for dim light. The cone cells have photopsin which is specialized for color. There is also another newly discovered pigment which is a non-visual pigment called melanopsin found in special ganglion cells. When melanopsin is activated, it triggers an entirely unique pathway that plays a significant role in resetting our biological rhythms.

This pathway goes to several important parts of our brain. The main destination is to the suprachiasmatic nucleus which is located in a tiny part of the center of brain called the hypothalamus which controls many of the most basic functions of the body like temperature and hunger. The suprachiasmatic nucleus synchronizes many clocks throughout our body. Remarkably, almost every cell in our body possesses a biological clock built into its DNA. These clocks need to be synchronized with the central clock in the brain. Morning sunlight plays a vital role in creating this synchronization throughout the body.

Light also affects the pineal gland which sits in the center of the brain and secretes a hormone called melatonin. Melatonin production is typically highest in darkness, signaling the body to prepare for sleep. For this reason it is often called the sleep hormone. Many people now take melatonin supplements to improve their sleep. Light has the effect of stopping melatonin production.

Another hormone involved in this early morning sunlight neurohack is cortisol, often known as the stress hormone. Cortisol is vital for numerous bodily functions. When we wake up in the morning, melatonin production ceases, and light acts as a stimulus to initiate cortisol release. Cortisol has been called the wakeful hormone because it helps stimulate the body in the morning.

When we don't experience morning light our biological rhythms can be disrupted. Individuals with desynchronized biological clocks often experience severe health problems. Night workers, for instance, face a myriad of issues affecting their cardiovascular and neurological health. They often experiencing depression. Seasonal affective disorder is another condition linked to disrupted biological rhythms and depression. It is observed in individuals living in northern climates during the winter when there is less light.

Uniqueness of Morning Sunlight

In the ancient science of Ayurveda, experiencing the morning sunlight (especially at sunrise) on a regular basis is considered highly beneficial for health. What is unique about the light at sunrise? The most obvious fact is that there is less white and blue light and more red and yellow. Additionally, near-infrared light, which is not visible is present at sunrise. Near-infrared light has been extensively studied for its therapeutic effects.

Light can also influence our body not only by interacting with the pigments in our eyes but by interacting and penetrating the skin. Vitamin D, of course, is produced by sunlight and has many beneficial effects on the body. There is a field of light therapy called red-light therapy which is also known as low-level light therapy (LLLT) and photobiomodulation (PBM therapy). Red light (630 to 660 nm) and near infrared (NIR) (810 to 850 nm) light can increase ATP production in our mitochondria, stimulate cerebral blood flow, cause the regrowth of neurons (a process called neurogenesis), and positively affect certain neurological and psychiatric disorders.

An oncologist in England, Dr. Mohammad Muneeb Khan, has suggested that early morning sunlight has another effect. He believes that this light penetrates our skin, enters our cells, and stimulates the mitochondria in the cells to produces melatonin. This cellular melatonin has a different function than the melatonin from the pineal gland. It acts as a powerful antioxidant that help protect the cells from wear and tear and aging.

In summary, morning sunlight has many beneficial effects. It enters our eyes and synchronizes our biological clocks, in part by stopping melatonin production. Morning sunlight also penetrates our skin and helps produce Vitamin D and also cellular melatonin which has an anti-aging effect. The growing body of research on the different effects of light therapy aligns with the ancient knowledge of Ayurveda and validates the importance of morning sunlight.

Starting Your Sunlight Habit

How can you incorporate more sunlight into your daily life? Use the Habit Map and Plan to see if you can make this a daily habit. Identify your main intention or desire as "getting more sunlight". Around this central goal, list at least three actions. Keep in mind that if you live in an area with limited sunlight, you can use alternative light sources like a ring light or full spectrum lamp. Think creatively about how to achieve your goal.

Next, consider the cue or prompt that will remind you to take action. For example, if you have dogs, your cue might be their morning walk routine. You can use this time to go outside with them and catch the sunrise. Alternatively, you could set an alarm as your cue, reminding yourself to step outside for 5 to 20 minutes during lunchtime to enjoy the natural light.

To measure your success, pay attention to how you feel after incorporating more sunlight into your routine. Additionally, you can keep a log or mark it on a calendar to track your progress and ensure you're consistently getting enough light exposure.

Lastly, don't forget to reward yourself. After a week or two of successfully adding more sunlight to your life, celebrate your achievement with a reward that will motivate you to continue.

NEUROHACK MAP & PLAN

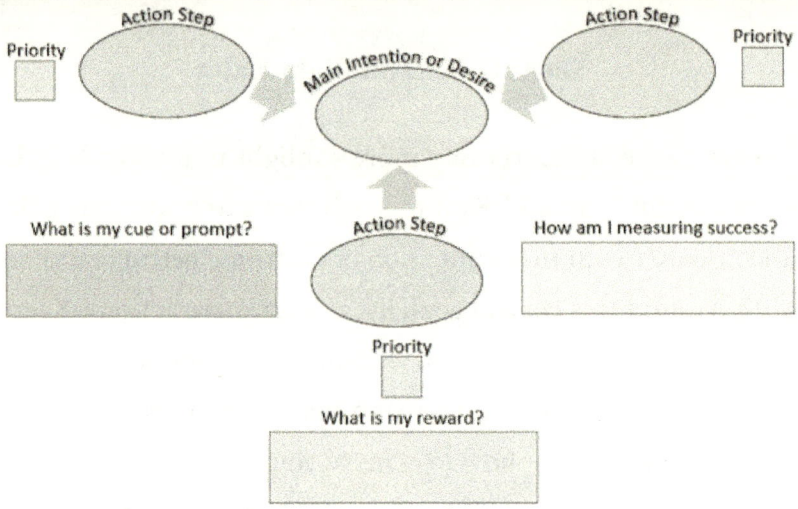

Priority

Action Step

Main Intention or Desire

Action Step

Priority

Action Step

Priority

What is my cue or prompt?

How am I measuring success?

What is my reward?

CHAPTER 8

BE REAL

The key to success is to genuinely recognize what you have accomplished with your neurohacks. By being real, you can assess your progress accurately and make meaningful adjustments to further enhance your neurohacks. Remember, the goal is personal growth and improvement, and that can only be achieved through sincere self-reflection and evaluation.

Celebrate your successes and identify areas where you can continue to grow. By embracing this "be real" approach, you will foster a deeper understanding of yourself and your capabilities, paving the way for continued personal development beyond the scope of this book.

How can you effectively evaluate the changes you've made? There are a few ways to approach this. First, you can use objective measures. For example, if you're aiming to lose weight, you can track your progress by regularly stepping on a scale. Similarly, if you want to assess your academic performance, you can rely on your grades as an objective measure. Keeping a log of your time spent on meditation practice allows you to monitor your consistency and progress in that area. Objective measures provide a clear and straightforward way to gauge your advancement.

In addition to objective measures, you can also evaluate your progress subjectively. This involves reflecting on your personal experiences, emotions, and overall sense of well-being. Subjective assessment may be more nuanced, while objective measures offer a simpler approach. By combining both objective and subjective evaluation methods, you can gain a comprehensive understanding of your progress.

Why does this assessment matter? It's essential because if you're not making the desired progress, you may need to make changes or explore alternative approaches. Regular evaluation allows you to determine whether the new habit you've implemented is effective or if it requires modification. By staying mindful of your progress, you can make informed decisions about your strategies and ensure you're on the right track toward achieving your goals.

In my own life, I (Carol) always believe in setting goals and having something to work toward. While a goal may not always be explicitly written on my calendar, its always in my mind. However, it's important to note that perfection should not be the ultimate aim. Instead, the goal should be to be the best version of yourself. Throughout these exercises, we've aimed to teach you how to personalize your plan so that it suits your current needs and enables you to become the best you can be.

Active Questions

Marshall Goldsmith, a renowned coach and author of the popular book *Triggers*, suggests that the best way to evaluate yourself is through the active question, "Did I do my best?" Although the book is primarily utilized in the business community, its principles are applicable to everyone. Goldsmith emphasizes the importance of framing questions in a way that holds individuals accountable for their actions.

For example, when you ask someone if they performed a particular habit or task, simply inquiring whether they did it today may elicit excuses and external justifications for why they did not complete it. However, the question, "Did you do your best to do this habit today?" shifts the focus to personal effort and eliminates external excuses. This approach encourages individuals to reflect on their level of commitment and the extent to which they prioritize the habit.

By adopting the active question approach, individuals are more likely to take ownership of their actions and make a genuine effort to fulfill their commitments. Positive accountability helps promote personal responsibility, leading to greater self-awareness and progress toward desired goals. The key question we're addressing here is about your level of motivation. Were you truly motivated or not? If not, why not? Do you really have other priorities? Our ultimate aim is to help individuals achieve full motivation and the ability to give their best effort in everything they do.

4 Levels of Feedback

In the book *Total Brain Coaching* Keith and his oldest son Ted Wallace developed the Feedback Matrix which is a tool that uses 4 levels of feedback from:

- Self-coaching

- Personal coaching

- Group coaching

- Environment coaching

Self coaching is the first level of feedback, where you maintain a journal or use a journaling app. In your journal, you objectively assess your progress and reflect subjectively on how well you are doing. This may require some extra effort, but it provides a clear record of your progress and valuable insights for improvement.

Let's consider Brianna, who decided as her first action step to review assignments in advance. If her chosen action step doesn't turn into a habit, she needs to try some of her other ideas like making sure she is practicing regular Transcendental Meditation or creating dedicated homework time. With each of her experiments she needs to both keep a record of the progress and include her thoughts about what is creating success or failure.

The second level of feedback comes from Personal coaching. It can be helpful to have a buddy who can check in with you and see how you are doing. We have already talked about having a buddy to work with and how using active questions can help you sustain your habits. If you can get the use of a professional coach that would be ideal. The coach can help you identify what goals and milestones you want to achieve. Most coaches will give you an idea of what is going to happen in the coaching sessions beforehand, and establish a code of conduct. The goal of the coach is help you find a solution and very often they will ask "What do you want to achieve by the end of our 45-minute session today?" Changing a habit often requires time, energy, and outside help.

The third type of feedback comes from Group coaching which can be in person or online. Working with a group can be very reinforcing. You can see how others are coping with the challenges of sticking with a new habit. Sometimes it is valuable to have other Energy State types in the group to create a livelier interaction.

The fourth and final type of feedback is through Environmental coaching. We might imagine ourselves as being independent of our environment, but this is generally not the case. We have talked about the importance of creating an ideal environment that will help minimize distractions and improve your focus on completing your homework assignments.

Neurohacking the Learning Cycle

In summary, we have introduced you to the concept of neurohacking and how it relates to your learning cycle. By understanding how you absorb knowledge best, you can enhance your skills significantly.

We have explored various ways to identify your learning style: visual, auditory, kinesthetic, or Ayurveda-based with a V, P, or K Energy State. Remember, there is no right or wrong type; it simply reflects how you learn best. Once you have identified your preference, it's crucial to tailor your educational experiences accordingly.

Let's recap the four components of the neurohack learning cycle. First, we have *Motivation*, which we've discussed as a critical aspect of learning. Fear is one aspect that can drive us to learn. The fear of falling behind or not meeting deadlines is a genuine concern. Life can also present obstacles, such as a sick child, which may limit the time available for studying. In such cases, it's important to collaborate with teaching assistants and instructors to find alternative solutions. Take responsibility for your situation and explore different approaches to meet the requirements within the given framework. Continuously strive to improve your learning by leveraging the tools and techniques that align with your unique style.

The most powerful motivation often comes from inspiration. Research consistently demonstrates that when individuals are inspired, they enjoy the learning process because they strive to become the best version of themselves. This is the key to success. Falling behind makes schoolwork more difficult, but by taking responsibility, staying proactive, and drawing on inspiration, you can navigate the challenges of online learning. Collaborate with your instructors and approach your studies through a mindset of inspiration rather than fear.

The second component is to *Personalize*. Carol experienced a tremendous improvement in her learning when she realized that she was a visual learner. She used to struggle with understanding content from video lectures, but by enabling closed captions, she found the material much easier to comprehend. In contrast, her husband was more auditory. We need to recognize that each individual is unique.

We've consistently highlighted the significance of *Experiment*, emphasizing that there are no right or wrong choices, only opportunities for learning. Without experimenting, we limit our ability to learn and grow.

In this chapter we have explored the concept *Be Real*, which involves assessing our progress honestly. If our current approach is not yielding the desired results, it's important to be open to switching to a new program or strategy. By being adaptable and willing to make adjustments, we increase our chances of success in the learning process.

Carol also shared a valuable lesson from her wonderful father, "Turning the Page." When faced with something that causes anxiety, simply turn the page. Take a moment to calm down, go for a walk, or take a deep breath. You'll discover that this approach can benefit you in various ways.

We have also emphasized the importance of breaking down your goals down into smaller, manageable neurohacks that you will enjoy doing. You will inevitably encounter assignments with multiple daunting steps, which can trigger anxiety. However, if you have learned how to focus on just one item at a time, tackling each step individually, you can systematically complete the entire assignment and also eliminate the anxiety that could overwhelm you. Don't view a large textbook as an insurmountable challenge, simply break it down into smaller sections.

We have learned that when transforming a neurohack into a habit it helps to have a trigger that prompts the start of your desired action. For example, Mondays could be the trigger. Every time Monday rolls around, it can serve as a reminder to begin your study routine. We have also learned that it's beneficial to incorporate a reward system. For some people, the reward could be the satisfaction of submitting assignments on time but for others it might mean going out and really celebrating.

Dopamine

Now, let's delve into what happens in the brain when a neurohack becomes a habit and you start feeling good about it. Dopamine is a neurotransmitter that plays an important role in the brain's reward system and our motivation cycle. Some refer to America as the "Dopamine Nation" because various addictive behaviors, including social media addiction, are driven by this neurotransmitter. Interestingly, it's not the pleasure itself that causes an increase in dopamine, but rather anticipation of the pleasure. For instance, the excitement of discovering an intriguing video or content keeps us engaged on social media platforms. Addiction and habits heavily rely on this neurotransmitter, as we actively seek experiences that boost our dopamine levels.

Understanding this system is essential, and if we examine the brain's different areas, we can identify the nucleus accumbens and the ventral tegmental area as key regions where dopamine is active. These areas, situated in the center of the brain, play a significant role in rewarding and motivating us, sometimes leading to unhealthy addictions. However, we can harness this powerful system to our advantage.

Instead of being trapped in old habits, we can replace them with new neurohacks that excite and interest us while promoting our well-being. By finding personalized, healthy neurohacks that align with our individual preferences, we can utilize the dopamine reward system to create positive anticipation and enjoyment. Whether it's practicing meditation, taking a walk in the sunlight, maintaining a healthy diet, or completing homework on time, we can leverage this dopamine system to reinforce positive behaviors and enhance our overall learning experience.

Conclusion

Take advantage of practices that have stood the test of time, such as Transcendental Meditation and yoga. These techniques are backed by scientific evidence. It remains your responsibility to apply and implement these practices in your life. At times, you may encounter periods of discomfort or imperfection in your experiences. In such situations, seek guidance, for example by attending group meditation sessions or consulting TM teachers, to reset and realign your neural circuits. These techniques are extremely effective, provided they are applied correctly. Remember that every aspect of life offers opportunities for improvement and advancement.

Despite developing learning agility, you will still encounter obstacles on your journey toward obtaining your goals. For example, pursuing a degree is a long process, and numerous life events may attempt to hinder your progress. However, winners overcome these hurdles. They view each obstacle as a challenge and seek ways to succeed, learning how to navigate past these obstacles.

In this context, a small failure is seen as an opportunity to learn and grow. No matter what happens, it's important to take responsibility and avoid playing the victim. Embrace the idea that whatever occurs is part of the learning process. Acknowledge its occurrence, and extract wisdom from it. The mindset we aim to cultivate is continuous learning. Stay focused on your goals and achieve everything you desire, both in your degree program and in your life. We wish you success on your journey to becoming the best possible version of yourself.

ABOUT THE AUTHORS

DR. ROBERT KEITH WALLACE

Dr. Robert Keith Wallace completed pioneering research on the Transcendental Meditation technique. His seminal papers on a fourth major state of consciousness—published in *Science, American Journal of Physiology,* and *Scientific American*—support a new paradigm of mind-body medicine and total brain development. Dr. Wallace was the founding President of Maharishi International University and has traveled around the world giving lectures at major universities and institutes, and has written and co-authored several books. He is presently a Trustee of Maharishi International University and Chairman of the Department of Physiology and Health.

CAROL PAREDES

Carol embarked on a transformative journey from a thriving technology career to a profound dedication to health and wellness. With an impressive track record of over 30 years in the technology field and a remarkable achievement of graduating summa cum laude with a B.S. in Software Development, Carol's expertise and passion have become a guiding light in her chosen path.

Today, Carol stands as an accomplished Ayurvedic Practitioner, Certified Integrative Nutrition Health Coach, and Yoga instructor, sharing her wealth of knowledge and nurturing well-being in the serene states of Maryland and Delaware. Her unwavering commitment to promoting holistic living has become the cornerstone of her life's purpose.

In March 2020, Carol's journey took an exciting turn as she joined the Physiology and Health Department at Maharishi International University. She earned her M.S. in Maharishi AyurVeda and Integrative Medicine in June of 2020.

Presently, Carol assumes the role of Associate Chair of the department, effortlessly blending her profound expertise in technology and wellness. With her unique perspective, she guides and inspires others on transformative journeys toward holistic living, illuminating the path to well-being and self-discovery. Carol's unwavering dedication and ability to combine diverse fields have positioned her as a beacon of wisdom and empowerment in her noble pursuit of promoting holistic well-being.

ACKNOWLEDGMENTS

Our deep appreciation goes to our very talented friend—George Foster for his outstanding cover design.

We would also like to thank Nicole Windenberger for excellent suggestions, editing, and proofreading.

REFERENCES

Chapter 1

The Power of Habit: Why We Do What We Do in Life and Business by Charles Duhigg, Random House, 2012

An Introduction to Transcendental Meditation: Improve Your Brain Functioning, Create Ideal Health, and Gain Enlightenment Naturally, Easily, Effortlessly by Robert Keith Wallace, PhD, and Lincoln Akin Norton, Dharma Publications, 2016

Transcendental Meditation: A Scientist's Journey to Happiness, Health, and Peace, Adapted and Updated from The Physiology of Consciousness: Part 1 by Robert Keith Wallace, PhD, Dharma Publications, 2016

Travis FT and Shear J. Focused attention, open monitoring and automatic self-transcending: Categories to organize meditations from Vedic, Buddhist and Chinese traditions. Consciousness and Cognition 19(4):1110-1118, 2010

Wallace RK. Physiological effects of Transcendental Meditation. Science 167:1751-1754, 1970

Wallace RK, et al. A wakeful hypometabolic physiologic state. American Journal of Physiology 221(3): 795-799, 1971

Wallace RK. Physiological effects of the Transcendental Meditation technique: A proposed fourth major state of consciousness. Ph.D. thesis. Physiology Department, University of California, Los Angeles, 1970

Schneider RH, et al. Stress Reduction in the Secondary Prevention of Cardiovascular Disease: Randomized, Controlled Trial of

Transcendental Meditation and Health Education in Blacks. Circ Cardiovasc Qual Outcomes 5:750-758, 2012

Rainforth MV, et al. Stress reduction programs in patients with elevated blood pressure: a systematic review and meta-analysis. Current Hypertension Reports 9:520–528, 2007

Brook RD, et al. Beyond Medications and Diet: Alternative Approaches to Lowering Blood Pressure. A Scientific Statement from the American Heart Association. Hypertension 61(6):1360-83, 2013

Cooper MJ, et al. Transcendental Meditation in the management of hypercholesterolemia. Journal of Human Stress 5(4): 24–27, 1979

Orme-Johnson DW and Walton KW. All approaches of preventing or reversing effects of stress are not the same. American Journal of Health Promotion 12:297-299, 1998

Barnes VA, et al. Impact of Transcendental Meditation on cardiovascular function at rest and during acute stress in adolescents with high normal blood pressure. Journal of Psychosomatic Research 51: 597-605, 2001

Jevning R, et al. Adrenocortical activity during meditation. Hormonal Behavior 10(1):54-60, 1978

Paul-Labrador M, et al. Effects of randomized controlled trial of Transcendental Meditation on components of the metabolic syndrome in subjects with coronary heart disease. Archives of Internal Medicine 166:1218-1224, 2006

Alexander CN, et al. Treating and preventing alcohol, nicotine, and drug abuse through Transcendental Meditation: A review and statistical meta-analysis. Alcoholism Treatment Quarterly 11: 13-87, 1994

Orme-Johnson DW, Herron RE. An Innovative Approach to Reducing Medical Care Utilization and Expenditures. American Journal of Managed Care 3: 135–144, 1997

Herron RE. Can the Transcendental Meditation Program Reduce the Medical Expenditures of Older People? A Longitudinal Cost-Reduction Study in Canada. Journal of Social Behavior and Personality 17(1): 415–442, 2005

Wallace RK, et al. The effects of the Transcendental Meditation and

TM-Sidhi program on the aging process. International Journal of Neuroscience 16: 53-58, 1982

Glaser JL, Brind JL, Vogelman JH, Eisner MJ, Dillbeck MC, Wallace RK, Chopra D, Orentreich N. Elevated serum dehydroepiandrosterone sulfate levels in practitioners of the Transcendental Meditation (TM) and TM-Sidhi programs. J Behav Med. 1992 Aug;15(4):327-41. doi: 10.1007/BF00844726. PMID: 1404349.

Alexander CN, et al. Transcendental Meditation, mindfulness, and longevity. Journal of Personality and Social Psychology 57: 950-964, 1989

Alexander CN, et al. The effects of Transcendental Meditation compared to other methods of relaxation in reducing risk factors, morbidity, and mortality. Homeostasis 35: 243-264, 1994

Schneider RH, et al. Long-term effects of stress reduction on mortality in persons > 55 years of age with systemic hypertension. American Journal of Cardiology 95: 1060-1064, 2005

Duraimani S, et al. Effects of Lifestyle Modification on Telomerase Gene Expression in Hypertensive Patients: A Pilot Trial of Stress Reduction and Health Education Programs in African Americans. PLOS ONE 10(11): e0142689, 2015

Wenuganen S, Walton KG, Katta S, Dalgard CL, Sukumar G, Starr J, Travis FT, Wallace RK, Morehead P, Lonsdorf NK, Srivastava M, Fagan J. Transcriptomics of Long-Term Meditation Practice: Evidence for Prevention or Reversal of Stress Effects Harmful to Health. Medicina (Kaunas) 57(3): 218, 2021

Alexander CN, et al. Transcendental Meditation, self-actualization, and psychological health: A conceptual overview and statistical meta-analysis. Journal of Social Behavior and Personality 6: 189-247, 1991

Eppley KR, et al. Differential effects of relaxation techniques on trait anxiety: A meta-analysis. Journal of Clinical Psychology 45: 957-974, 1989

Alexander CN, et al. Effects of the Transcendental Meditation program on stress-reduction, health, and employee development: A prospective study in two occupational settings. Stress, Anxiety and Coping 6: 245–262, 1993

Harung HS, et al. Peak performance and higher states of consciousness:

A study of world-class performers. Journal of Managerial Psychology 11(4): 3–23, 1996

Nidich S, et al. Non-trauma-focused meditation versus exposure therapy in veterans with post-traumatic stress disorder: a randomised controlled trial. Lancet Psychiatry 5(12):975-986, 2018

Dr Andrew Huberman, Neurobiologicist and Associate Professor at Stanford interviewed by Rich Roll at https://www.youtube.com/watch?v=SwQhKFMxmDY

Chapter 2

Atomic Habits: An Easy & Proven Way to Build Good Habits & Break Bad Ones by James Clear, Avery, 2018

Cook DA, Artino AR Jr. Motivation to learn: an overview of contemporary theories. Med Educ. 2016 Oct;50(10):997-1014. doi: 10.1111/medu.13074. PMID: 27628718; PMCID: PMC5113774.

Morris LS, Grehl MM, Rutter SB, Mehta M, Westwater ML. On what motivates us: a detailed review of intrinsic v. extrinsic motivation. Psychol Med. 2022 Jul;52(10):1801-1816. doi: 10.1017/S0033291722001611. Epub 2022 Jul 7. PMID: 35796023; PMCID: PMC9340849.

Simon Oliver Sinek is a British-born American author and inspirational speaker. He is the author of five books, including *Start With Why*. His Ted talk can be seen at: https://www.ted.com/talks/simon_sinek_how_great_leaders_inspire_action/c?language=en

Chapter 3

Childs-Kean L, Edwards M, Smith MD. Use of Learning Style Frameworks in Health Science Education. Am J Pharm Educ. 2020 Jul;84(7):ajpe7885. doi: 10.5688/ajpe7885. PMID: 32773837; PMCID: PMC7405309.

Stander J, Grimmer K, Brink Y. Learning styles of physiotherapists: a systematic scoping review. BMC Med Educ. 2019 Jan 3;19(1):2. doi:

10.1186/s12909-018-1434-5. PMID: 30606180; PMCID: PMC6318981.

Vidal PP, Lacquaniti F. Perceptual-motor styles. Exp Brain Res. 2021 May;239(5):1359-1380. doi: 10.1007/s00221-021-06049-0. Epub 2021 Mar 6. PMID: 33675378; PMCID: PMC8144157.

http://www.educationplanner.org/students/self-assessments/learning-styles.shtml

Chapter 4

Living in Balance with Maharishi AyurVeda: Practical Therapies for Consciousness-Based Health by Robert Keith Wallace, PhD, Karin Pirc, MD, Julia Clarke, MS

Wallace, R.K. Ayurgenomics and Modern Medicine. Medicina 2020, 56, 661

Wallace, RK. The Microbiome in Health and Disease from the Perspective of Modern Medicine and Ayurveda. Medicina 2020; 56, 462.

Chapter 5

Total Brain Coaching: A Holistic System of Effective Habit Change For the Individual, Team, and Organization by Ted Wallace, MS, Robert Keith Wallace, PhD, and Samantha Wallace, Dharma Publications, 2020

Self Empower: Using Self Coaching, Neuroadaptability, and Ayurveda by Robert Keith Wallace, PhD, Samantha Wallace, Ted Wallace, MS, Dharma Publications, 2021

Wallace, R.K.; Wallace, T. Neuroadaptability and Habit: Modern Medicine and Ayurveda. Medicina 2021, 57, 90. doi: 10.3390/medicina 57020090

16 Super Biohacks for Longevity: Shorcuts to a Healthier, Happier, Longer Life by Robert Keith Wallace, PhD, Ted Wallace, MS, Samantha Wallace, Dharma Publications, 2023

Chapter 6

Gut Crisis: How Diet, Probiotics, and Friendly Bacteria Help You Lose Weight and Heal Your Body and Mind by Robert Keith Wallace, PhD, Samantha Wallace, Dharma Publications, 2017

The Rest And Repair Diet: Heal Your Gut, Improve Your Physical and Mental Health, and Lose Weight by Robert Keith Wallace, PhD, Samantha Wallace, Andrew Sternberg, MA Jim Davis, DO, and Alexis Farley, Dharma Publications, 2019

Lee DH, Rezende LFM, Joh HK, Keum N, Ferrari G, Rey-Lopez JP, Rimm EB, Tabung FK, Giovannucci EL. Long-Term Leisure-Time Physical Activity Intensity and All-Cause and Cause-Specific Mortality: A Prospective Cohort of US Adults. Circulation. 2022 Aug 16;146(7):523-534. doi: 10.1161/CIRCULATIONAHA.121.058162. Epub 2022 Jul 25. PMID: 35876019; PMCID: PMC9378548.

Mu X, Liu S, Fu M, Luo M, Ding D, Chen L, Yu K. Associations of physical activity intensity with incident cardiovascular diseases and mortality among 366,566 UK adults. Int J Behav Nutr Phys Act. 2022 Dec 13;19(1):151. doi: 10.1186/s12966-022-01393-y. PMID: 36514169; PMCID: PMC9745930.

Wang Y, Nie J, Ferrari G, Rey-Lopez JP, Rezende LFM. Association of Physical Activity Intensity With Mortality: A National Cohort Study of 403 681 US Adults. JAMA Intern Med. 2021 Feb 1;181(2):203-211. doi: 10.1001/jamainternmed.2020.6331. PMID: 33226432; PMCID: PMC7684516.

Sanders LMJ, Hortobágyi T, Karssemeijer EGA, Van der Zee EA, Scherder EJA, van Heuvelen MJG. Effects of low- and high-intensity physical exercise on physical and cognitive function in older persons with dementia: a randomized controlled trial. Alzheimers Res Ther. 2020 Mar 19;12(1):28. doi: 10.1186/s13195-020-00597-3. PMID: 32192537; PMCID: PMC7082953.

Aguib Y, Al Suwaidi J. The Copenhagen City Heart Study (Østerbroundersøgelsen). Glob Cardiol Sci Pract. 2015 Oct 9;2015(3):33. doi: 10.5339/gcsp.2015.33. PMID: 26779513; PMCID: PMC4625209.

Atakan MM, Li Y, Koşar ŞN, Turnagöl HH, Yan X. Evidence-Based Effects of High-Intensity Interval Training on Exercise Capacity and

Health: A Review with Historical Perspective. Int J Environ Res Public Health. 2021 Jul 5;18(13):7201. doi: 10.3390/ijerph18137201. PMID: 34281138; PMCID: PMC8294064.

Booth, FW; Roberts, C.K; Laye, M.J. Lack of exercise is a major cause of chronic diseases. Compr. Physiol. 2012, 2, 1143–1211

Hallal, PC. Andersen, L.B.; Bull, F.C.; Guthold, R.; Haskell, W.; Ekelund, U. Global physical activity levels: Surveillance progress, pitfalls, and prospects. Lancet 2012, 380, 247–257.

Bull, FC; Al-Ansari, SS; Biddle, S; Borodulin, K; Buman, MP; Cardon, G.; Carty, C.; Chaput, JP.; Chastin, S.; Chou, R.; et al. World Health Organization 2020 guidelines on physical activity and sedentary behaviour. Br. J. Sports Med. 2020, 54, 1451–1462.

Paluch AE, Gabriel KP, Fulton JE, et al. Steps per Day and All-Cause Mortality in Middle-aged Adults in the Coronary Artery Risk Development in Young Adults Study. *JAMA Netw Open.* 2021;4(9):e2124516. doi:10.1001/jamanetworkopen.2021.24516

Sleiman SF, Henry J, Al-Haddad R, El Hayek L, Abou Haidar E, Stringer T, Ulja D, Karuppagounder SS, Holson EB, Ratan RR, Ninan I, Chao MV. Exercise promotes the expression of brain derived neurotrophic factor (BDNF) through the action of the ketone body β-hydroxybutyrate. Elife. 2016 Jun 2;5:e15092. doi: 10.7554/eLife.15092. PMID: 27253067; PMCID: PMC4915811.

Cooney GM, et al. Exercise for depression. JAMA. 2014;311:2432.

Peterson DM. The benefits and risks of exercise. https://www.uptodate.com/contents/search. Accessed Sept. 15, 2017.

Greer TL, et al. Improvements in psychosocial functioning and health-related quality of life following exercise augmentation in patients with treatment response but nonremitted major depressive disorder: Results from the TREAD study. Depression and Anxiety. 2016;33:870.

Schuch FB, et al. Exercise as treatment for depression: A meta-analysis adjusting for publication bias. Journal of Psychiatric Research. 2016;77:42.

Zschucke E, et al. Exercise and physical activity in mental disorders: Clinical and experimental evidence. Journal of Preventive Medicine and Public Health. 2013;46:512.

Anderson E, et al. Effects of exercise and physical activity on anxiety. Frontiers in Psychiatry. 2013;4:1.

Isaac AR, Lima-Filho RAS, Lourenco MV. How does the skeletal muscle communicate with the brain in health and disease? Neuropharmacology. 2021 Oct 1;197:108744. doi: 10.1016/j.neuropharm.2021.108744. Epub 2021 Aug 5. PMID: 34363812

Saeed SA, Cunningham K, Bloch RM. Depression and Anxiety Disorders: Benefits of Exercise, Yoga, and Meditation. Am Fam Physician. 2019 May 15;99(10):620-627. PMID: 31083878.

Wang WL, Chen KH, Pan YC, Yang SN, Chan YY. The effect of yoga on sleep quality and insomnia in women with sleep problems: a systematic review and meta-analysis. BMC Psychiatry. 2020 May 1;20(1):195. doi: 10.1186/s12888-020-02566-4. PMID: 32357858; PMCID: PMC7193366.

Groessl EJ, Liu L, Chang DG, Wetherell JL, Bormann JE, Atkinson JH, Baxi S, Schmalzl L. Yoga for Military Veterans with Chronic Low Back Pain: A Randomized Clinical Trial. Am J Prev Med. 2017 Nov;53(5):599-608. doi: 10.1016/j.amepre.2017.05.019. Epub 2017 Jul 20. PMID: 28735778; PMCID: PMC6399016.

Arendt J. Melatonin: Countering Chaotic Time Cues. Front Endocrinol (Lausanne). 2019 Jul 16;10:391. doi: 10.3389/fendo.2019.00391. PMID: 31379733; PMCID: PMC6646716.

Poza JJ, Pujol M, Ortega-Albás JJ, Romero O; Insomnia Study Group of the Spanish Sleep Society (SES). Melatonin in sleep disorders. Neurologia (Engl Ed). 2022 Sep;37(7):575-585. doi: 10.1016/j.nrleng.2018.08.004. Epub 2020 Sep 18. PMID: 36064286.

Bueno APR, Savi FM, Alves IA, Bandeira VAC. Regulatory aspects and evidences of melatonin use for sleep disorders and insomnia: an integrative review. Arq Neuropsiquiatr. 2021 Aug;79(8):732-742. doi: 10.1590/0004-282X-ANP-2020-0379. PMID: 34550191.

Besag FMC, Vasey MJ, Lao KSJ, Wong ICK. Adverse Events Associated with Melatonin for the Treatment of Primary or Secondary Sleep Disorders: A Systematic Review. CNS Drugs. 2019 Dec;33(12):1167-1186. doi: 10.1007/s40263-019-00680-w. PMID: 31722088.

Reiter RJ, Ma Q, Sharma R. Melatonin in Mitochondria: Mitigating Clear and Present Dangers. Physiology (Bethesda). 2020 Mar

1;35(2):86-95. doi: 10.1152/physiol.00034.2019. PMID: 32024428.

Melhuish Beaupre LM, Brown GM, Gonçalves VF, Kennedy JL. Melatonin's neuroprotective role in mitochondria and its potential as a biomarker in aging, cognition and psychiatric disorders. Transl Psychiatry. 2021 Jun 2;11(1):339.

Li T, Jiang S, Han M, Yang Z, Lv J, Deng C, Reiter RJ, Yang Y. Exogenous melatonin as a treatment for secondary sleep disorders: A systematic review and meta-analysis. Front Neuroendocrinol. 2019 Jan;52:22-28. doi: 10.1016/j.yfrne.2018.06.004. Epub 2018 Jun 15. PMID: 29908879.

Foley HM, Steel AE. Adverse events associated with oral administration of melatonin: A critical systematic review of clinical evidence. Complement Ther Med. 2019 Feb;42:65-81. doi: 10.1016/j.ctim.2018.11.003. Epub 2018 Nov 3. PMID: 30670284.

Scholtens RM, van Munster BC, van Kempen MF, de Rooij SE. Physiological melatonin levels in healthy older people: A systematic review. J Psychosom Res. 2016 Jul;86:20-7. doi: 10.1016/j.jpsychores.2016.05.005. Epub 2016 May 10. PMID: 27302542.

Culpepper L, Wingertzahn MA. Over-the-Counter Agents for the Treatment of Occasional Disturbed Sleep or Transient Insomnia: A Systematic Review of Efficacy and Safety. Prim Care Companion CNS Disord. 2015 Dec 31;17(6):10.4088/PCC.15r01798. doi: 10.4088/PCC.15r01798. PMID: 27057416; PMCID: PMC4805417.

Zare Elmi HK, Gholami M, Saki M, Ebrahimzadeh F. Efficacy of Valerian Extract on Sleep Quality after Coronary Artery bypass Graft Surgery: A Triple-Blind Randomized Controlled Trial. Chin J Integr Med. 2021 Jan;27(1):7-15. doi: 10.1007/s11655-020-2727-1. Epub 2021 Jan 8. PMID: 33420602.

Murray BJ, Cowen PJ, Sharpley AL. The effect of Li 1370, extract of Ginkgo biloba, on REM sleep in humans. Pharmacopsychiatry. 2001 Jul;34(4):155-7. doi: 10.1055/s-2001-15876. PMID: 11518478.

Djokic G, Vojvodić P, Korcok D, Agic A, Rankovic A, Djordjevic V, Vojvodic A, Vlaskovic-Jovicevic T, Peric-Hajzler Z, Matovic D, Vojvodic J, Sijan G, Wollina U, Tirant M, Thuong NV, Fioranelli M, Lotti T. The Effects of Magnesium - Melatonin - Vit B Complex Supplementation in Treatment of Insomnia. Open Access Maced J Med Sci. 2019 Aug

30;7(18):3101-3105. doi: 10.3889/oamjms.2019.771. PMID: 31850132; PMCID: PMC6910806.

Sutanto CN, Loh WW, Kim JE. The impact of tryptophan supplementation on sleep quality: a systematic review, meta-analysis, and meta-regression. Nutr Rev. 2022 Jan 10;80(2):306-316. doi: 10.1093/nutrit/nuab027. PMID: 33942088.

Dasdelen MF, Er S, Kaplan B, Celik S, Beker MC, Orhan C, Tuzcu M, Sahin N, Mamedova H, Sylla S, Komorowski J, Ojalvo SP, Sahin K, Kilic E. A Novel Theanine Complex, Mg-L-Theanine Improves Sleep Quality via Regulating Brain Electrochemical Activity. Front Nutr. 2022 Apr 5;9:874254. doi: 10.3389/fnut.2022.874254. PMID: 35449538; PMCID: PMC9017334.

Fetveit A, Skjerve A, Bjorvatn B. Bright light treatment improves sleep in institutionalised elderly-an open trial. Int J Geriatr Psychiatry. 2003 Jun;18(6):520-6. doi: 10.1002/gps.852. PMID: 12789673.

Higuchi S, Motohashi Y, Liu Y, Maeda A. Effects of playing a computer game using a bright display on presleep physiological variables, sleep latency, slow wave sleep and REM sleep. J Sleep Res. 2005 Sep;14(3):267-73. doi: 10.1111/j.1365-2869.2005.00463.x. PMID: 16120101.

Kanda K, Tochihara Y, Ohnaka T. Bathing before sleep in the young and in the elderly. Eur J Appl Physiol Occup Physiol. 1999 Jul;80(2):71-5. doi: 10.1007/s004210050560. PMID: 10408315.

Youngstedt SD, Kripke DF, Elliott JA. Is sleep disturbed by vigorous late-night exercise? Med Sci Sports Exerc. 1999 Jun;31(6):864-9. doi: 10.1097/00005768-199906000-00015. PMID: 10378914.

Chapter 7

Hamblin MR. Photobiomodulation for Alzheimer's Disease: Has the Light Dawned? Photonics. 2019 Sep;6(3):77. doi: 10.3390/photonics6030077. Epub 2019 Jul 4. PMID: 31363464; PMCID: PMC6664299.

Montazeri K, Farhadi M, Fekrazad R, Akbarnejad Z, Chaibakhsh S, Mahmoudian S. Transcranial photobiomodulation in the management of brain disorders. J Photochem Photobiol B. 2021 Aug;221:112207. doi:

10.1016/j.jphotobiol.2021.112207. Epub 2021 May 5. PMID: 34119804.

Do MTH. Melanopsin and the Intrinsically Photosensitive Retinal Ganglion Cells: Biophysics to Behavior. Neuron. 2019 Oct 23;104(2):205-226. doi: 10.1016/j.neuron.2019.07.016. PMID: 31647894; PMCID: PMC6944442.

Lazzerini Ospri L, Prusky G, Hattar S. Mood, the Circadian System, and Melanopsin Retinal Ganglion Cells. Annu Rev Neurosci. 2017 Jul 25;40:539-556. doi: 10.1146/annurev-neuro-072116-031324. Epub 2017 May 17. PMID: 28525301; PMCID: PMC5654534.

Barolet D, Christiaens F, Hamblin MR. Infrared and skin: Friend or foe. J Photochem Photobiol B. 2016 Feb;155:78-85. doi: 10.1016/j.jphotobiol.2015.12.014. Epub 2015 Dec 21. PMID: 26745730; PMCID: PMC4745411

Reiter RJ, Tan DX, Rosales-Corral S, Galano A, Zhou XJ, Xu B. Mitochondria: Central Organelles for Melatonin's Antioxidant and Anti-Aging Actions. Molecules. 2018 Feb 24;23(2):509. doi: 10.3390/molecules23020509. PMID: 29495303; PMCID: PMC6017324.

Reiter RJ, Ma Q, Sharma R. Melatonin in Mitochondria: Mitigating Clear and Present Dangers. Physiology (Bethesda). 2020 Mar 1;35(2):86-95. doi: 10.1152/physiol.00034.2019. PMID: 32024428.

Melhuish Beaupre LM, Brown GM, Gonçalves VF, Kennedy JL. Melatonin's neuroprotective role in mitochondria and its potential as a biomarker in aging, cognition and psychiatric disorders. Transl Psychiatry. 2021 Jun 2;11(1):339. doi: 10.1038/s41398-021-01464-x. PMID: 34078880; PMCID: PMC8172874.

Reiter RJ, Sharma R, Pires de Campos Zuccari DA, de Almeida Chuffa LG, Manucha W, Rodriguez C. Melatonin synthesis in and uptake by mitochondria: implications for diseased cells with dysfunctional mitochondria. Future Med Chem. 2021 Feb;13(4):335-339. doi: 10.4155/fmc-2020-0326. Epub 2021 Jan 5. PMID: 33399498.

Engel KW, Khan I, Arany PR. Cell lineage responses to photobiomodulation therapy. J Biophotonics. 2016 Dec;9(11-12):1148-1156. doi: 10.1002/jbio.201600025. Epub 2016 Jul 8. PMID: 27392170.

Srivastava AK, Roy Choudhury S, Karmakar S. Near-Infrared Responsive Dopamine/Melatonin-Derived Nanocomposites Abrogating in Situ Amyloid β Nucleation, Propagation, and Ameliorate Neuronal Functions. ACS Appl Mater Interfaces. 2020 Feb 5;12(5):5658-5670. doi: 10.1021/acsami.9b22214. Epub 2020 Jan 27. PMID: 31986005.

Reiter RJ, Sharma R, Rosales-Corral S. Anti-Warburg Effect of Melatonin: A Proposed Mechanism to Explain its Inhibition of Multiple Diseases. Int J Mol Sci. 2021 Jan 14;22(2):764. doi: 10.3390/ijms22020764. PMID: 33466614; PMCID: PMC7828708.

Dr Andrew Huberman, Neurobiologicist and Associate Professor at Stanford talks about the value of sunlight: https://www.youtube.com/watch?v=yBjUR16AiBMD

Chapter 8

Triggers: Creating Behavior That Lasts—Becoming the Person You Want to Be by Marshall Goldsmith and Mark Reiter, Crown Business, 2015

Index

sunrise 71, 73, 74, 75
suprachiasmatic nucleus 72

T

TM v, 1, 2, 3, 26, 55, 86, 95
Transcendental Meditation v, 1, 11, 12, 18, 26, 41, 55, 61, 85, 89, 93, 94, 95
Turning the Page 7, 8, 9, 10, 12, 83

V

Vata 42, 43, 44, 47, 63, 65, 67, 68
V Energy State 43, 49, 55, 56, 58, 63, 65, 67
visual learners 30
vitamin D 74

Y

Yoga 65, 100

www.ingramcontent.com/pod-product-compliance
Lightning Source LLC
Chambersburg PA
CBHW031130020426
42333CB00012B/315